The D.I.Y. Diet

Janet Menzies

The D.I.Y Diet

FOURTH ESTATE
LONDON

First published in Great Britain in 1995 by
Fourth Estate Limited
289 Westbourne Grove
London W11 2QA

A catalogue record for this book is available from the British
Library.

ISBN 1–85702–219–X

Typeset by York House Typographic Ltd, London
Printed in Great Britain by Cox & Wyman Ltd, Reading, Berks.

To my husband

Contents

PART ONE

Introduction: The Terrible Truth About Diets

There is an awful secret about dieting. The terrible truth about dieting is that 90 per cent of all diets fail.

Yes, it's true. Most professional nutritionists, diet researchers and many health writers have known this for some time. On the face of it this is pretty dreadful news for you, reading this book and wanting to succeed, and for me, wanting to prove that this book has been worth your buying. Here we are, the two of us, facing the sad fact that we've only a 10 per cent chance of winning. In fact, if I don't do something about it fast I won't be able to succeed at all, because even if you and 9 of your determined friends are successful in your diets, what about the other 90 readers who could soon be chucking this book in the bin as yet another useless diet book?

I've spent the last eight years mulling this problem over, ever since I discovered the truth about diets while researching an article on health myths for the *Daily Mail*. When I began my research the first thing I came up with was a lot more questions that had to be answered. I wanted to know why we all keep going on all these diets and buying diet products if nine times out of ten we find it a complete waste of effort and money.

The answer is obvious. Like an explorer looking for the North West Passage, we won't give up looking until we find what we are searching for – in our case a diet that succeeds. And of course there is a whole multi-million pound diet industry out there, dedicated to encouraging our quest with more and more spurious claims and false promises.

Even more importantly, though, I wanted to know what was different about those 10 per cent of diets that do succeed. Was it something special about the dieters – were they superhuman, ultra-disciplined beings for whom temptation knew no power? In that case, how had they got into the position of having to go on a diet in the first place?

Or was it the diet that was so magical? Was it the real answer at last, the philosopher's stone of diets that could turn all leaden flesh into gold-tanned muscle? Again, if that was the case, nobody would have kept that particular diet secret and we'd all be on it, and no doubt someone would be making a fortune out of having invented it.

Common sense told me that neither of those provided the answer. Everybody knows you can't turn base metal into gold, and there's no North West Passage. So I looked again at the whole issue of dieting. First of all the 90 per cent. What do we mean by failure of a diet?

Speaking to diet organisations and health researchers, I discovered that a diet can fail in two major ways:

- The first way is one many of us are familiar with: the dieter does not achieve the goal weight. This happens either through giving up before the diet has run its course (no, honestly, if it wasn't for work I really could have done that poached salmon *en croûte* three times a day diet); or because the dieter completes the prescribed duration of the diet, but still doesn't lose the desired amount of weight.

- The second way occasionally makes newspaper headlines. This is when a dieter achieves the goal weight and then puts most or even all of the weight back on again once off the prescribed diet regime.

I suspect that for most of us a combination of these two factors is at work. We always have a goal weight a couple of pounds lower than we ever achieve, and when we finish a diet the weight seems to creep back on again. The result is usually much the same. We go out and buy the next best-selling diet that comes along and off we all go again.

Once I knew the two types of diet failure, I wanted to know why they occur. I started by looking at the diets themselves. I read hundreds of different diets – some only a few hundred words long, some the length of a small novel. And I discovered another very strange truth. With only a few exceptions these diets were all excellent in terms of nutrition and general health principles.

Yes! Nearly all these diets that weren't working were actually jolly sound. They were based mainly on the nutritional commandments of reduced calories, low fat, low sugar, high fibre, medium protein, plenty of fruit and vegetables, which doctors know to be good for humans. The only thing I could find wrong with any of them was that they demanded a great deal of commitment to follow them precisely. There was a level of weighing, measuring, advance preparing and special shopping involved that I really couldn't see anybody managing on a regular basis without hired help. Certainly any averagely busy person with a job, a family, a house and even a very quiet social life to run would give up after a few days unless they were completely obsessive. For example, there was one that required fresh fish every other night – all well and good if you finish work in time to get to a fishmonger (what's a fishmonger, Mummy?) on your way home. So I concluded that one of the problems with diets is that they usually demand too great a degree of commitment from the dieter.

That couldn't be the whole answer though. People – researchers and dieters alike – have complained of this fact for some time now, and I certainly wasn't the first to work it out. In fact there is a new generation of diets about at the moment which tries to do away with calorie-counting altogether. Yet diets are still failing – so although this is part of the answer it can't be the whole solution.

Ironically it was while adapting extracts from one of these new wave diets for newspaper publication that I stumbled on the real reason diets fail. In an effort to abandon calorie-counting this diet gave all foods ratings based on how good they were for you. If a food was bad for you it was given a minus rating. In theory all you had to do for the diet to succeed was eat plenty of high rated foods and few minus rated foods so that at the end of each day you achieved the right rating overall.

Fine as far as it goes, but the ratings given to some foods were totally arbitrary. Because there had recently been a great deal written about calcium deficiencies the diet's author had rated milk extremely high. Meanwhile my husband had just been told his severe kidney stones were being caused by calcium in his diet, and if he was to avoid further serious kidney problems he must give up all calcium-containing foods at once.

My husband will not mind me letting slip that, at this period, he was definitely overweight. If, in the quest to lose those surplus pounds, he had unwittingly followed the recommendations of the diet, and eaten those high rated foods, he would have been taking in what were for him dangerously high levels of calcium. For him that diet, in general terms nutritionally sound, would have been the equivalent of taking poison. I was aghast! The diet didn't explain what nutritional content it was that was giving a food a high rating, nor did it have any warnings about dieters with special requirements. The diet would have been fine for me, and I could easily have suggested it to my husband. If I had done so I would have been condemning him to the repeated agony of kidney stones – just ask anybody who's ever had one what the pain is like.

Thank heavens I know the nutritional composition of most foods, but what about the majority of dieters who don't have that sort of specialist knowledge? Even as I sighed with relief for having spotted the diet's booby trap, I suddenly knew that I had stumbled across the fundamental problem with diets: what is right for one dieter may not be right for another.

My husband's is an extreme case, of course, but it gave me the clue I needed to work out the reason diets fail: that what's good for one person may be quite bad for another. Heard it somewhere before? Yes: one man's meat is another man's poison. The more I thought about it the more I could see that the diet which might fit in perfectly with one person's requirements, perhaps for high fibre, might be full of problems for another dieter – someone with an irritable bowel, for example.

And then I realised: one person's healthy slimming diet is somebody else's recipe for disaster. But each diet book tells us all to go on the *same* diet. It is so simple. Not all dieters are the same, but every new diet demands that all dieters follow it, and only it.

It's true isn't it? What best-selling diet have you ever seen that suggested the next diet book on the newsagent's shelf might work better for you than it could? What diet have you ever seen that even acknowledged that there *could* be any other way of losing weight?

I had discovered not only why 90 per cent of diets fail, but also why a mysterious 10 per cent succeed. Probably by complete coincidence, that 10 per cent of successful dieters had happened to strike on the diet that was right for them. This truth was so basic and so startling that I immediately decided to stop researching other people's diet books and writing about them for newspapers, and instead broadcast my discovery: *all dieters are different, so they should follow different diets*.

The more I thought about it and researched it, the more sense it made. We are all different in shape, size, personality, habits. We don't all do the same jobs, have the same clothes, share the same lifestyles, so why ever should we be brainwashed into thinking we must all follow the same diet? You'd be furious if

someone wrote a much-hyped book telling you what car to drive
and what television programmes to watch, and you certainly
wouldn't buy the book, no matter how many millions of copies it
sold. So why on earth buy a book telling you to eat the same as
everybody else? . . . Because you are desperate to lose a bit of
weight.

Well, that's no reason to lose your common sense as well. You
may want or need to diet, but that doesn't stop you being an
individual, and as an individual your diet requirements will be
different from other people's. That's why this diet is called the
D.I.Y. Diet – because it gives you the alternatives from which to
make your own personal choice. So read on to find out how the
D.I.Y. Diet works, and how you can make it part of your life.

How the D.I.Y. Diet Works

Conventional diets fail in 90 per cent of cases for two reasons:

- They dictate the same diet for all dieters, regardless of their
  different situations.
- They demand too great a degree of commitment from the
  dieter.

The D.I.Y. Diet answers both these problems:

- The D.I.Y. Diet provides a series of D.I.Y. eating plans
  which meet the personal requirements of individual dieters.
- The D.I.Y. Diet uses alternative and substitute foods instead
  of requiring calorie-counting and portion-sizing. This
  makes it much easier for the dieter to make it part of a
  long-term lifestyle. The D.I.Y. Diet has 11 different eating
  plans. You choose the particular eating plan that is right
  for you.

The next section of the D.I.Y. Diet is devoted to helping you choose the right diet, and showing you how easy it is to follow.

Starting the D.I.Y. Diet

Diets always seem confusing, and are often impossible to follow, because they dictate the same programme for everybody. In fact we all have completely individual physiques and metabolisms, just as we have individual personalities. No diet can work for you if it is contrary to your metabolic personality. The D.I.Y. Diet has 11 different eating plans, each one suited to a different metabolic group. This section shows you how to discover your metabolic personality. First, you have to find out exactly which eating plan to choose. To help you do this I have borrowed a technique used by computer programmers, called a flow chart, to produce a map with questions about your body at each of the major junctions. All you have to do is follow this Eating Plans Map (pp. 12–13), taking the No or Yes route at each question box, and you will eventually end up at your destination – the correct eating plan for you.

When you are following the map you may want to rush ahead and answer Yes to more than one of the major junction boxes. Resist this. The Eating Plans Map is designed to help you arrive at your most important problem first.

For example, when using the Eating Plans Map you may answer Yes to the question 'Are you overfat everywhere?' and you would therefore arrive immediately at the Low-calorie Eating Plan. At the same time you may feel you also have bingeing problems or high blood pressure, which would call for a different diet plan. The answer is not to lose your common sense. First things first. Let's deal with this overfat problem, and when you have succeeded in that we will see whether you still have the bingeing and blood pressure problems. In many cases you will find that simply losing your excess fat, and the mixed emotions this inspires, helps you with your bingeing problem. And of course the first thing doctors recommend for overfat people with high blood pressure is loss of excess fat. If you have succeeded with the Low-calorie Eating Plan, but still have bingeing problems or high blood pressure, the answer is simple. Just follow the Eating Plans Map again, this time taking the bingeing route.

Fat and Weight Are Not The Same

From now on you will not read the phrases 'overweight' or 'weight loss' in this book. There is no such thing as an overweight body. A body's weight is what it weighs, neither more nor less than that. There is nothing intrinsically better about a body that weighs 8 stone than a body that weighs 10 or 15 stone.

Fat is the problem, not weight, and fat is not weight. In fact fat is actually quite light – certainly when compared with muscle. Instead of the term 'overweight' I use 'overfat'. If you weigh more than somebody else of your height you don't necessarily have a problem, but if you are carrying excess fat on your body, you need to reduce the amount of fat on your body to somewhere nearer the norm.

EATING PLANS MAP

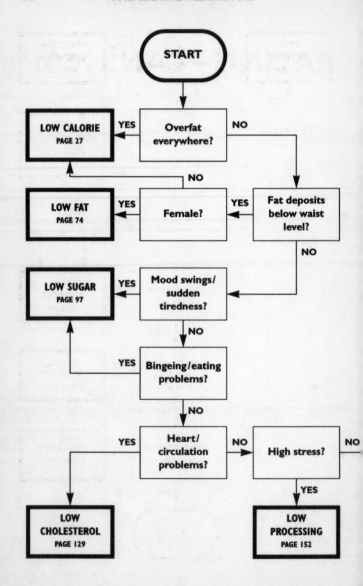

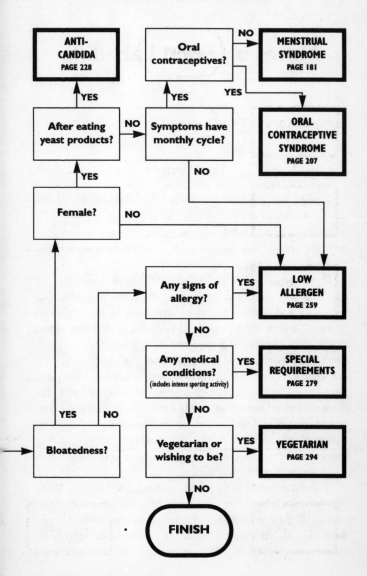

Notes on Food Labelling

Label Lunacy

Time and again in this book you will be urged to read the label of any food product you buy so that you will know exactly what is in it. This is easier said than done. Marketing men want you to buy their product and they are not too scrupulous in the methods they use to attract you.

In the past, highly processed foods were a novelty and nutrition was taken for granted, so the marketing men used gimmicks and bright colours to attract us to buy. 'Instant', 'purified' and 'ready to eat' were regarded as excellent selling points to emphasise on a food product's label. Today there is much more awareness of nutrition. Since the late 70s and early 80s there have been successive fads for low-calorie, wholemeal, unprocessed, high-fibre, low-cholesterol and low-fat foods. The marketing men have rapidly latched on to these nutrition crazes and have labelled their foods accordingly to emphasise any traits a particular food may have that matches the current trend. Any element of the same food that does not accord with the nutrition trend is simply not highlighted.

A classic example is the labelling of breakfast cereals. When first marketed, breakfast cereal was basically a packet of pre-cooked flaked or puffed grains flavoured with sugar and salt and fortified with vitamins. The nature of the basic ingredients meant that breakfast cereal was low in fat and contained reasonable amounts of dietary fibre and vitamins but was relatively high in salt and sugar. It was a fairly neutral foodstuff, neither especially bad nor especially good for you, though useful in mass catering and as a method of vitamin supplementation. A century later the composition of breakfast cereal remains *exactly the same*. But in the intervening years it has been marketed in all these different ways:

- A health food conducive to bowel management (Swiss muesli).
- A morally purifying food (turn-of-the-century America).
- A nutritious source of energy (Force wheat flakes: 'Force is the force that raises him').
- A wonderful way to get children to eat vitamins (with the introduction in the 50s of novelty cereals aimed specifically at children).
- A low-calorie breakfast (Special K).
- A great source of bran fibre (with the popularity of Audrey Eyton's F-Plan Diet).
- A natural food without artificial additives (at the height of the food colourings scare).
- Rich in glucose for energy (in the Steve Cram commercial for Start, and the only instance I can think of where marketing has actually advertised the fact that breakfast cereal is high in sugar).
- A quick way to prepare food (during the fast-food 80s).
- A way of reducing blood cholesterol (at the height of the popularity of oats).
- A food with comforting overtones of childhood nostalgia (the recent Kelloggs cornflakes commercial aimed at 30-somethings who were the first children to have novelty cereals and now have children of their own).
- A food that is low in fat (the actual slogan is 'low in fat, and always has been').

Any historian could find a fascinating chronology of our changing social and health preoccupations just through looking at the marketing of one single foodstuff that has not changed its nutrition attributes for about 100 years.

The point is that the marketing men want you to think breakfast cereal is constantly new and different, and always the right food for you no matter what the fad of the moment is. So the fact that breakfast cereal is highish in sugar and salt is not mentioned, because these are not currently regarded as beneficial, but attributes that cereal happens to have by coincidence (like being low in fat, as every grain product is) are emphasised.

This happens with almost any processed and packaged foodstuff you care to look at. Thus a tin of baked beans in the 80s would have sold itself to you as being recommended by the F-plan Diet, but today it will stress that it is low in fat. In neither case is the fact emphasised that baked beans are fairly high in sugar and salt (the fourth and fifth highest percentage ingredient respectively).

Reading Labels

So how is the consumer to fight her way through all this misleading gimmickry in order to find out exactly what a specific product's nutritional qualities are?

Here are some simple rules.

• **Take nothing for granted**
Just because it says 'free from artificial colour and preservative' in big letters doesn't mean it is also free of other nutritional nasties.

• **Read the small print**
Manufacturers are legally obliged to list all the ingredients of the product. Don't look at all the advertising spiel, look where it says INGREDIENTS . . .

● **First is most**

By convention nearly all lists of ingredients name the highest quantity ingredient first and so on in descending order to the smallest quantity. So if sugar is the first mentioned ingredient then the product contains more sugar than it does any other single ingredient – even though the product may be called 'Original recipe healthy tomato sauce' rather than 'Sugar and water sauce with added flavouring'. Funny that, isn't it!

● **Ignore aliases**

These days many manufacturers fight shy of talking about sugar. Instead they will mention malt (basically a sugar derived from barley), glucose, fructose, syrup, brown sugar, demerara sugar, molasses, natural raw cane sugar, treacle. But when it gets into the body it's all just sugar. Watch out for similar weasel words for salt, flavourings, etc.

● **Check portion size**

Many products list calories and other nutritional elements in 'amount per serving'. If they want you to think it is low-calorie, the portion size mentioned will be about half what you would regard as a normal portion. If they want you to think it is rich in fibre and trace elements then the portion size mentioned will be far more than you could face at a single sitting. So once in a while weigh or measure out the portion size they mention on the pack and then you'll see what we are really talking about.

● **Get to know your percentages**

The best way round the portion problem is to look at the nutritional analysis per 100 grams. Most of the more enlightened manufacturers list this in addition to the amount per portion. By looking at the 100 gram guide you get an instant picture of what percentage of the product each different nutritional element provides. Because it is expressed in x grams per 100 grams you have a simple way of knowing the percentage. For example, on a baked beans tin 13 grams carbohydrate per 100 grams means that the product, baked beans, contains 13 per cent carbohydrate.

Now check your eating plan to see how much carbohydrate you should be eating and you can see whether it falls within the limits.

For example, it is recommended that we eat no more than 30 per cent fat in our diet. If we check the label of every food we eat and none of it is more than 30 per cent fat, we know that no matter how much we eat, we are not getting more than 30 per cent fat. This assumes we always eat labelled food and never eat a food like butter which is more than 30 per cent fat, but all the same, it's a jolly useful guideline.

● **Trust only figures**

When it comes to the section of the label marked 'nutrition information' or 'nutritional analysis' the manufacturers must be totally factual. Look closely at these figures and make sure you understand what is meant by the various nutritional elements mentioned. This is the only place on the label where you can't be misled by marketing hype.

● **Become a label cynic**

Whenever you see some wonderful claim on the label of a food, distrust it immediately. All marketing men are guilty until proven innocent. Just check out the list below to see the many wonderful ways they have to bamboozle you.

Words They Use on Labels

Normal people are brought up to assume that labelling something is a way of conveying information about that object. But to a marketing man the label is his last and best chance of getting you to buy the product. So he will manipulate the information on the label in order to make the product as appealing as possible. Label language falls into three basic categories:

1 Pure hype: meaningless muddling words intended to con you into thinking well of the product.
2 Half truths: information that is basically accurate but presented in a misleading way.
3 Genuine information: factual truth that means exactly what it says.

Pure Hype: Marketing Men's Meaningless Muddlers

Depending on current consumer trends and values, and the nature of the product, the types of phrases used will fall into various categories designed to elicit different positive emotions in the consumer. Have you ever fallen for any of these?

● **The Feel-Good Factor**

COUNTRY, FARM FRESH, FARMHOUSE, FARM LAID: Designed to make you feel secure and appeal to your nostalgic impulses. The reality behind these phrases is that there is nothing special about food grown in the country or on a farm. Where else would food come from? The farming countryside is after all just one massive food production factory. Don't confuse 'farm laid' with free range either: 'farm laid' means 'battery farmed' as sure as eggs are eggs.

GENUINE, LUXURY, MEATY, ORIGINAL, PREMIUM, SPECIAL, TRADITIONAL: Emphasising traditional 'olde worlde' values, these phrases are what the marketing men call 'positive value reinforcers'. They make you feel as if you are buying something of proven quality and integrity without actually making any real promises. The words are deliberately woolly and subjective. Anything that isn't a forgery is genuine, whether it's genuine junk food or what. Meaty need only mean that the product contains a fraction of meat to pass the Trades Descriptions Act.

And all premium means is pricey. For an acid test, just try putting the words into a proper sentence: 'original . . . as opposed to what?'

● **The Health Kick**

BROWN, FIBRE ENRICHED, FULL OF NATURAL GOODNESS, HEALTHY, NUTRITIOUS: After the boring rationed food of the war years the consumer wanted novelty in food, so in the 50s and 60s marketing men would never have dreamt of stressing the health aspects even of a food that was genuinely highly nutritious. But since we have all become so preoccupied with healthy eating these attributes are now seen as very marketable. Again the phrases used are deliberately vague and unquantifiable. Brown isn't always better, for example, there is no nutritional difference between brown sugar and white sugar. Since it is indigestible, fibre cannot nutritionally speaking enrich a food. Natural doesn't necessarily mean good – what is good anyway? All food is good for your health to the extent that it keeps you alive. If it's a digestible, edible food then it is nutritious (i.e. containing nutrient) and that still includes the sugar, the fat, and the cholesterol.

● **The Green Theme**

HOME-GROWN, HOME-MADE, HOME-STYLE, HERITAGE, NATURAL, ENVIRONMENT FRIENDLY, GREEN, PURE: The environmental movement has had a wide-ranging impact on our thinking in the 90s, but much of its influence is emotional and arbitrary. An excellent example is the way marketing men have exploited our innocent desire to do what is best for our families and our planet. Once again using words which it would be very difficult to prove were lies, the marketing man nevertheless gives the consumer the impression that by buying the product she is doing her bit. In the context of food production 'home' can mean anything from a huge factory (with a live-in night watchman) to an unsanitary private kitchen. Natural is simply an all-encompassing phrase to which our society happens to attach positive emotions: sugar is natural; fat is natural but that doesn't mean you should eat it. Pure is also a specious phrase: all it actually means is that the product is unadulterated – it doesn't preclude it from being unadulterated junk.

Half-truths

CONSERVATION GRADE APPLIED FOR: All well and good, but it doesn't mean they've got it, does it?

DIET: Most uses of this word genuinely mean that the food is either calorie-free or significantly lower in calories than the non-diet version of the food. However, a diet version of a very high-calorie food could still be quite high in calories.

GLUCOSE: Another version of sugar.

HIGH IN POLYUNSATURATES: But polyunsaturate fats are still fats. This food is not guaranteed to be low in calories, nor is it guaranteed to be low in saturated fats – it could have lots of both types of fat.

HIGH-FIBRE: Contains a reasonable amount of roughage, but may also contain a high amount of sugar, fat and artificial additives – they're making no promises about those.

LITE/LIGHT: Vague term used to suggest that the product is lower in calories and/or fat than normal versions. The phrase is often abused, so you need to check the ingredients label closely.

LONG-LIFE: Treated or packaged in such a way as to prevent rapid deterioration. Need not be a bad thing but can be a hint of additives and high processing.

LOW-CALORIE: Significantly lower in calories than the ordinary version of the product, but not guaranteed to contain fewer than a specific number of calories. Low-calorie crisps are still relatively high in calories compared with a carrot. Ironically carrots cannot be labelled low-calorie because there isn't a higher calorie version of a carrot!

LOW-FAT: As with calories, really means lower-fat rather than low in absolute terms.

MALT/MALTY: Barley sugar. Watch out for 'malty goodness' – a real case of double speak.

NATURAL SWEETENING: Sugar.

NO ARTIFICIAL COLOURINGS: Does not contain manufactured chemically derived colouring agents, but may contain naturally derived colours including caramel and carotin.

NO ARTIFICIAL FLAVOURS: Does not contain manufactured chemical seasonings but may contain sugar, salt and many other naturally occurring flavours.

NO PRESERVATIVES: If the product also has a long shelf-life, be very suspicious of this claim. Even sugar is a preservative, and for food to be kept from spoiling it is necessary for there to be some sort of preserving process, even if it is only freezing.

ORGANIC: Should mean more than it does. The phrase was abused during the 80s health food boom. Today trading standards officers are trying to enforce the use strictly. Genuinely organic food should have a Soil Association label.

SUGAR-FREE: But not necessarily free from artificial sweeteners. If you want something sweet to eat take your pick, but don't kid yourself that you get sweetness without paying a nutritional price.

Genuine Information

BARN LAID: The hens which laid the eggs live together in a barn (fairly crowded but not battery).

CONSERVATION GRADE: Has been raised and farmed according to standards laid down by the Soil Association. Conservation grade meat has been reared eating strictly monitored foodstuff.

DO NOT RE-FREEZE: Means the product has been frozen once already.

FREE RANGE: Hens living outdoors with roosts and nest boxes available.

GLUTEN-FREE: Not containing any wheat element, suitable for allergics and coeliacs.

OPEN FARMED: Means the animal was reared outdoors with shelter available.

SOIL ASSOCIATION APPROVED: Organically grown according to the rules of the Soil Association.

SUITABLE FOR VEGETARIANS: Contains no animal product.

Spaghetti Shapes with Meatballs in Tomato Sauce

FREE FROM ARTIFICIAL COLOUR AND PRESERVATIVE

What it means
does not contain any manufactured chemicals, but almost certainly contains sugar

Ingredients:
tomatoes, pasta shapes (made from wheat), burgers (contains colour – caramel), sugar, flour, salt, modified corn-flour, herbs, citric acid, spices, cheese.
Minimum 12% meat.

What it means
ingredients are usually (but not always) listed in order of quantity with the largest first, so tomatoes may be the main ingredient in this product. Note, sugar is likely to be the fourth highest quantity ingredient. Caramel is a burnt sugar used to brown meat. Citric acid is a preservative derived from lemon juice.

Nutrition Information:
Typical values per 200g serving (half can)

energy	175kcal
protein	7.9g
carbohydrate	24g
(of which sugars	10.2g)
fat	5.3g
(of which saturates	2.3g)
fibre	1.4g
sodium	0.9g

What it means
175 calories; 4% protein; 7% complex carb; 5% refined carb; 1% unsaturated fat; 1% saturated fat; 0.7% fibre; 0.5% salt
What it does not say
what the other 80.8% is; why a minimum of 12% meat only provides a maximum of 4% protein.
Does it make nutritional sense?
Not very much. Sugar content is rather high and fibre low, but fat is within guidelines.

PART TWO
THE EATING PLANS

1. The Low-calorie Eating Plan

LOW-CALORIE PLAN CHECK CHART

Before you start the Low-calorie Eating Plan, fill in the check chart below by ticking any Yes answers to double-check that you have chosen the most appropriate eating plan.

1.	Last year's clothes are too small.	☐
2.	Friends have commented on my loss of figure.	☐
3.	My face seems to have lost definition.	☐
4.	I know I have been eating too much.	☐
5.	My size has increased evenly everywhere.	☐
6.	I can pinch rolls of fat over ribs, under shoulder blades, at backs of arms and over hips.	☐
7.	I can pinch rolls of fat over hips but not elsewhere.	☐
8.	I feel generally healthy and I am not pregnant.	☐
9.	I have been fat more or less as long as I can remember.	☐
10.	I have trouble sticking to diets.	☐

Ticks KEY

0–3 The Low-calorie Eating Plan is not ideal for you. Look at the flow chart (pp. 12–13) again and try to be completely honest in your answers.

4–8 The Low-calorie Eating Plan will be right for you, but remember your requirements may change over the next few months.

9–10 You have additional eating needs which may mean other plans are

more suitable for you. If you have answered Yes to 7, you
should move straight on to the Low-fat Eating Plan (p. 74). If
you have answered Yes to 10, fill in the low-sugar check chart
(p. 97) and then make your own mind up which will work
best, or alternate between the two. If you answered Yes to 9,
read the section on congenital obesity (p. 53) before you
commence the Low-calorie Eating Plan.

IMPORTANT: If you did not answer Yes to 8, make sure there are
no medical reasons why you should not go on the Low-calorie
Eating Plan. You can check this with your family doctor. You
should also check the Special Requirements Eating Plan (p. 279).

WELCOME TO THE LOW-CALORIE EATING PLAN

Here is the good news: of all the eating plans in this book, the
basic low-calorie plan is the simplest and most straightforward
to follow, so you've got a head start already.

If you have dieted before you will recognise similarities
between the low-calorie plan and other diets you may have tried.
The plan also has similarities with other diets in this book. This is
because the Low-calorie Eating Plan is a general diet, suitable for
a wide range of people who have no other health, eating or
physical problems or circumstances apart from being or believing themselves to be generally overfat.

The Low-calorie Eating Plan represents much of the nutritional thinking expounded in the Nutritional Advisory Committee on Nutrition Education's ground-breaking report on diet in
1983. Though now more than a decade old, this famous
NACNE report still acts as a starting point for sensible thinking
on diet.

NACNE was one of the first bodies to confirm that calorie-counting was neither necessary nor indeed advisable for those who wished to decrease their overfat. Instead NACNE recommended that dieters should not reduce substantially the amount of food they ate, but should alter their eating habits to concentrate more on healthy foods.

It was from this basic, nutritionally sound idea that I developed the concept of substitution. Nearly every diet up until now has told you to eat less or deprive yourself in some way. I don't want you to deprive yourself for the rest of your life. All you have to do on any of the eating plans is move away from the foods which are not suitable for you and eat more of the ones which will be neutral or beneficial in effect. Once you have stabilised in achieving most of the goals in your eating plan, you can even begin to eat the unsuitable foods, as long as you do so in moderation.

Very few dieters would recognise this diet as being anything like the conventional slimming diets they have been used to, that is why I use the phrase eating plan. An eating plan abolishes all the negative aspects of slimming diets which we now know can be harmful. Unlike a conventional slimming diet, an eating plan has no constant calorie-counting; no repetitious weighing and measuring of portions and ingredients; and no faddy food rules.

Over the last five years we have come increasingly to recognise that conventional slimming diets not only do not work, but can have bad effects both nutritionally and psychologically. One of the worst problems of calorie-counting is that it tends to reinforce the very obsessive attitude to food that the idea of the diet was supposed to overcome. Put simply: when you eat too much you think about food a lot – when you go on a diet you think about food all the time.

Ultimately the only truly successful way to lose overfat permanently is for food to cease to be such an important factor in your life. That means the Low-calorie Eating Plan has to be easy to follow; being on it is not going to dominate your day.

To increase the chances of success to the maximum, the Low-calorie Eating Plan embraces the art of the possible. Instead of setting out with unrealistic goals and setting down ridiculously demanding rules, the Low-calorie Eating Plan embodies what is well within your scope to achieve. Let's be realistic. If a diet is going to require an immense amount of effort on your part, it is unlikely to be successful, and even if you succeed at first you'll find it hard to maintain.

We all lead busy lives and we have only so much energy. The fact of the matter is that our fat-loss programme really isn't the most important thing in our lives – it would be unhealthy if it was. For nearly all of us who have ever dieted, losing a bit of fat is not a matter of life and death and it's time we stopped treating it as if it was. In fact most of us fail in our conventional slimming diets because, thank heavens, we are sane enough not to treat them as a matter of life and death.

So for this eating plan to be successful it needs first and foremost to be possible. And that means accepting compromise right from the outset without blaming or punishing yourself for being less than perfect.

The whole concept of substitution is based on compromise. OK, you want a bar of chocolate. It's no good trying to tell yourself not only not to have a bar of chocolate but to have nothing at all. So have a substitute instead.

The substitute food may not be super-healthy itself, but for you personally it is probably less unhealthy than a bar of chocolate. Some of the time even the substitute won't do; it just has to be the bar of chocolate. But if you can limit those times, or decrease the amount of chocolate you eat when you do, then you're beginning to win. And, even more importantly, the battle is being won without too great a personal cost. To succeed permanently the eating plan aims to become part of your lifestyle without you even noticing. If the sacrifice required to reach a particular goal is too great, you either won't get there in the first place or won't stay when you've arrived.

As most dieters know, that is precisely the problem that leads to the dangerous syndrome of on-off dieting. Eat, drink and be merry, for tomorrow we diet, is the saying with which every slimmer is familiar. But if you are going to diet on 5 or 6 or however many tomorrows it also means you are going to binge on 5 or 6 or however many todays. You don't binge before starting the Low-calorie Eating Plan because you won't be denying yourself while you are on it, just changing the way you eat slightly.

If this is the first time you have attempted to lose excess fat, congratulations, because it will almost certainly be the last – and you won't have gone through all the previous rigours endured by on-off dieters.

If this is your first attempt because you have only recently become overfat, your chances of success are even greater. The body has a natural tendency to stabilise at a certain level of fatness, and if this has been fairly low for the majority of your life it will take little encouragement on your part to get the body to return to it.

Conversely, if your body has always had a tendency to be overfat, then it is more difficult for you to become permanently slim. Turn to the section on congenital obesity at the end of this chapter and you will find lots of helpful extra hints that could make the difference between success and failure.

HOW IT WORKS

The Low-calorie Eating Plan couldn't be simpler. Listed in the 'stop' lists are foods that for one reason or another will maintain your existing levels of fat. The main reason why these foods contribute to fat maintenance is because they are 'calorie-dense', that is, they have a greater number of calories contained in a relatively small volume of food.

A typical example of calorie-dense food is a cube of fat or a teaspoon of sugar, both of which contain far more calories than a carrot, yet the carrot is larger and more satisfying. Fibre and water are the main components that prevent a food from being calorie-dense, so the more fibrous and juicy the food, the more likely it is to be fairly low in calories.

The root of the Low-calorie Eating Plan is the idea that you should avoid calorie-dense foods as much as possible and substitute them with foods which are 'good value for calories' – that is, foods which offer emotional and physical satisfaction as well as nutritional content, without being too high in calories. Occasionally a food will be fairly calorie-dense, but will offer such good value for those calories that it should not be regarded as a 'stop' food – some meats and cheeses fit into this category.

Also there may be times when a 'stop' food becomes good value for calories because the need for it (emotional or otherwise) is so pressing. Before taking a food temporarily off your stop list for this reason, evaluate your thinking carefully. Work out if anything else (not necessarily food) would fulfil the same need (it might be a luxurious bath, for example); or whether a substitute food will do. If you still think you need the stop food, then have it.

But remember, each time you have that stop food you are decreasing your chances of success. So, as always in this book, aim for a compromise. Most of the time use the substitute food – that's what it's there for – and save the stop food for your time of greatest need (as the Good Witch would say). One trick is pretending you can have the stop food once and once only, and you have to work out which is the moment when it will have the greatest effect.

If you find you are resorting to a particular stop food constantly, then you should look at whether you might be a compulsive eater (see the Low-sugar Eating Plan, p. 97) or you might have an allergy/addiction syndrome (see the Low-allergen Eating Plan (p. 259)).

Or it may simply be that losing your overfat isn't important enough to you. If that's the case then work out what really is important to you and go for it.

Maybe you've decided to become slimmer because other areas of your life are unsatisfactory. Think hard about this, be honest with yourself, and do something about the real problem rather than going on another diet.

Another widespread reason why slimming diets fail is so logical that only Wonderland characters could refuse to believe it. It is because the slimmer is *already slim enough*. I know – heresy, isn't it? But consider this. If you've never been able to get below 8½ stone no matter how hard you diet, perhaps it's because that is the right weight for you.

Johnny Francome described how when he was a jockey he was having terrible trouble sticking to his riding weight. He ate little and spent hours in the sauna, but still his weight had a tendency to rise above the weight that he was advertised to racehorse trainers as being able to 'do'. The answer was simple, he said: 'I revised my riding weight.' So trainers were told that from now onwards the minimum weight at which Francome would be able to ride was several pounds heavier.

As soon as I heard that, I revised my 'riding weight' by nearly half a stone and have never looked back. If you have always had trouble shedding the notional last few pounds, I do advise you to 'revise your riding weight' – regardless of what it might say in the height/weight charts.

STEP-BY-STEP GUIDE TO THE LOW-CALORIE EATING PLAN

1. Read all sections of the diet carefully.
2. Learn what the stop foods are and why you must stop them.
3. Get familiar with all the substitutes and where to buy them.
4. Go through the week-long sample eating programme and work out how it will fit into your lifestyle.
5. If you are at all uncertain you can decide to follow the sample eating programme exactly for a week until you get the hang of things.
6. Learn how to make the snack substitutes and recipes.
7. Make a copy of the glance guide to stop and substitute foods.
8. Take the glance guide shopping with you to make sure you are stocking up on the right foods.
9. Remember that any food not mentioned as a stop food can be eaten whenever you like.
10. Note which drinks are to be stopped.
11. Eat plenty of fresh vegetables, these are not stop foods.
12. Follow the diet for 2 months before reviewing your symptoms and deciding whether to continue on it, change to another diet, or return to normal eating.

STOP, THINK, SUBSTITUTE

Which foods should I stop eating and what should I substitute?

Complex Carbohydrate Group

Complex carbohydrates do not present much of a problem for those following this general low-calorie eating plan because they are not 'calorie-dense'. That means that the calories are present along with a whole complex of other dietary ingredients including fibre, water, vitamins and even some protein. There-fore with each mouthful you are ingesting (taking in) a wide range of dietary ingredients, not just calories. Thus 'complex' carbohydrates are more filling and provide better nutritional value per calorie than refined carbohydrates.

Refined carbohydrates have been processed to remove the complex of ingredients and refine it down to just one thing – basically sugar – known as the 'refined' carbohydrate. Therefore 'refined' carbohydrates and products made from them are very calorie-dense. Because the other dietary factors like fibre, water, etc. have been stripped away, the same size mouthful contains far more calories for far less nutritional value than it does with a complex carbohydrate.

Complex carbohydrates are basically the so-called starchy foods – bread, flour, cereals, pasta, rice, potatoes. Provided you don't add calorie-dense products like sugar or fat to your complex carbohydrate food, the low-calorie plan eater is gener-ally OK to browse freely in this group. But to help your plan along it is probably a good idea to start by avoiding the more highly processed foods. A simple tip is to avoid 'white' carbo-hydrates like white bread, white rice and white flour. There's no particular reason to do this long-term – nutritionists recognise that non-wholegrain products do have their place in a balanced diet – but it will get you off to a flying start.

- **Stop**: White bread; muesli; white flour.

- **Substitute**: Granary bread; porridge or plain oat flakes; cornflour (instead of white flour and fat for thickening sauces).

Refined Carbohydrate Group

As we learnt in the section above, when you refine a complex carbohydrate what you get is basically a sugar. Sugar has been compared with cocaine – pure, white and deadly. In fact it is nothing of the sort. It is simply a source of calories. What exactly are calories anyway?

Calories are very simple. A calorie is the name we give to a unit of energy. When we are talking about nutrition the sort of calorie energy we are talking about is the energy that our bodies can use as fuel to maintain life functions.

In fact very many sources of heat-giving fuel are measured in calorific units, not just dietary calories. So there is nothing wrong with a calorie *per se*. As you know, animals (including humans) do in fact die quite rapidly without adequate calorie intake.

So if refined carbohydrate, that is sugar, is nothing but calories, and there is nothing wrong with calories, what can be wrong with sugar? The answer – the very fact that it is nothing but calories. This causes two problems:

1 Sugar is very calorie-dense, that is, a very small amount of it contains a comparatively high number of calories. This means that if it is eaten in the same volume as complex carbohydrates, an excess of calories can rapidly be ingested. It is very likely to be eaten in the same volume as complex carbohydrates because the stomach measures satisfaction more by simple volume than by calorific intake.

2 Sugar does not contain the complex range of other nutrients and dietary factors required for the body to function healthily. Therefore the fibre, water, vitamins, proteins and trace elements required must be obtained from other dietary sources where they will be present along with more calories. So if an eating pattern contains a high proportion of sugar calories, yet more calories will have to be ingested in order to obtain other vital nutrients.

It therefore makes much more sense to get value for your calories by eating foods that contain a combination of calories and nutrients all in one go.

In theory it should be possible to live on sugary foods alone, provided you take a full range of vitamin and mineral pills and protein tablets and eat a fair amount of cardboard. In reality this sort of science fiction space-man diet proves to be very unhealthy, especially for people who have problems metabolising sugar (see the Low-sugar Eating Plan, p. 97, for more information about this).

So most sensible low-calorie eating plans start from the principle that it is a good idea to reduce your intake of refined carbohydrates as much as possible and substitute complex carbohydrates instead. Indeed many people find they become less obese simply by taking this one easy measure.

- **Stop**: Anything with a high sugar content (sugar, syrup, treacle, malt – honey is permitted in small quantities); cakes; biscuits; pâtisserie (cream cakes, etc.); commercially manufactured foods high in sugar, e.g. puddings, desserts, breakfast cereals; croissants; doughnuts.

- **Substitute**: Variety breads (e.g. continental, rye, soda, granary, etc.) smeared with a trace of honey and plenty of cottage cheese (flavoured if desired) or 'diet' dairy products; crispbreads with savoury spreads; fresh fruit with 'diet' dairy products; oatcakes with yoghurt. Use fruit juice or honey for sweetening in cooking.

Protein Group

Like carbohydrates, proteins are an essential nutrient to humans. Proteins occur in a wide range of foods, including some plants and cereals as well as meat and fish. The body's digestion breaks protein down first into peptone and then into peptides, which are amino acids. These amino acids are used as the body's building blocks to create and repair tissue and other functions, including muscle, blood, etc.

Unlike carbohydrates, the amino acids are not used as a primary energy fuel. Think of the difference between using wood to make a fire and using wood to make a table and that's pretty much the difference between carbohydrate (firewood) and protein (carpentry timber). Just as you don't burn the table unless you've run out of firewood, so the body does not convert protein into fuel energy unless it has insufficient carbohydrate.

So for the low-calorie planner there ought to be no problem here, since the body will use your protein calories for other purposes than making you overfat. In fact for very many people there isn't one. But most of the conventional dietary patterns in the West happen to be very rich in protein – largely because we are wealthy enough to be able to afford it. So we tend to eat more protein than our body needs.

And what happens if you have got far more tables than you need? You might put them on the fire anyway along with the kindling. That is pretty much what the body does when it has more than enough protein to provide for bodily functions. It uses the protein as extra fuel, and on a low-calorie eating plan the last thing you need is spare fuel calories.

The other problem with protein in the wealthy Western diet is that our preferred source of protein is meat (again, the most expensive and difficult protein to produce), and most of this meat is fairly high in saturated animal fats. To compound the problem, the way in which Westerners prepare their meats for eating very often involves the addition of more fat in the shape of frying, roasting, etc.

Westerners tend to concentrate exclusively on meat for their protein source, rather than ingesting a wide range of dietary protein sources (e.g. rice, pulses, nuts, fish, cheese, eggs, soya bean curd). Unlike other dietary protein sources meat is not only very protein-rich, its fat is also very calorie-dense. So Westerners tend to eat more protein than their bodies need (especially with their sedentary lifestyles) and that protein also carries along with it an excess of calorie-dense fat, therefore too many calories as well.

Research has also indicated that fat carries its own health risks apart from obesity, and these are discussed under the fats section (p. 41).

Most nutritionists now agree that if Westerners were to do three things about dietary protein, their health and obesity problems would decrease. These are:

- Reduce the total proportion of protein in the diet.
- Obtain protein from a wider range of sources than just meat.
- Eat leaner meat or meat that is prepared in a low-fat way.

Again, many obesity problems have been solved just through adjusting these factors without taking any other dietary measures.

- **Stop:** Fatty meats and meat products with a high fat content (sausages, pork pies, Scotch eggs, etc.); fried meats and fried fish; rich, spicy meats; peanuts; taramasalata.

- **Substitute:** Fresh, low-processed meat and fish products; lean meats; grilled meat and fish; vegetarian products (including bean curd); pulses.

Vegetable and Fruit Group

The good news for low-calorie eating planners is that vegetables and fruit are essentially an excellent dietary source. Especially if eaten as fresh and with as little preparation as possible (and farmed chemical-free as far as possible), fruit and vegetables are an ideal source of dietary fibre, carbohydrate, vitamins and trace elements, at the same time as being generally low in calorie density.

The only problems that may arise are in the preparation of the fruit and vegetables. If they are overcooked or overstored they can lose nutritional value. If they are cooked in fat or oil they will become calorie-dense. However, in an otherwise well-balanced low-calorie eating plan, even frying vegetables occasionally is not a problem. Begin by avoiding calorie-dense cooking methods with your fruit and vegetables, but as your eating becomes better balanced and your overfat decreases you can afford to be less strict about it.

- **Stop:** Deep-fried vegetables (onion rings, breadcrumbed mushrooms, etc.); deep-fried fruit fritters; chips; roast potatoes; sugar-sweetened fruit juices and fruit products.

- **Substitute:** Shallow stir-fried vegetables (cut small to cook quickly); fresh raw and steamed vegetables and salads; baked, mashed or boiled potatoes; fresh fruit stewed in its own juice; unsweetened fruit juices.

Dairy Group

Nutritionists today are very much divided about dairy products. One school of thought points out that dairy products are calorie-dense and produced from animal fat – both of which we know to be dietary problems. But other nutritionists, especially recently, have pointed out that this is more than compensated for by the rich supply of calcium, vitamins and trace elements in dairy products. They also have the merit of not being very highly processed in an age where much of the food we ingest has been overprocessed.

I think it is very much a matter of personal habits. If you rarely drink much milk and without thinking confine yourself to just a scraping of butter on your toast then it doesn't really make much sense to worry unduly about your dairy intake. If, on the other hand, you are someone who can drink a pint of milk straight out of the fridge, cooks constantly with lashings of butter, and frequently browses on cheese, then dairy products are almost certainly contributing to your overfat problem. If you are honest with yourself you certainly know which of these you are, and if it is the latter, then adopt the stop/substitute regime.

- **Stop**: Full cream milk; butter; full cream dairy products (cream cheeses); chocolates; chocolate, malted and sweetened milk shake drinks.

- **Substitute**: Skimmed milk; low-fat spread; low-fat yoghurt and fromage frais (diet and flavoured versions permitted, without sugar); yoghurt and skimmed milk shakes sweetened with fruit purée or juice (or sugar substitute).

Fats Group

Not only are animal fats calorie-dense without providing a particularly good range of nutrients (though more than sugar), there is also evidence to suggest that animal 'saturated' fats pose a threat to health. The British Heart Foundation is now certain that a high saturated fat intake can contribute towards raising blood cholesterol levels, especially the 'bad' cholesterol, low-density lipoprotein (*LDL*). High blood cholesterol levels have for some time been associated with increased risk of arterial and cardiac (artery and heart) diseases.

But – and almost every nutrition story has two sides – the latest research now tends to pinpoint genetic factors (inherited from your parents) as playing a greater part in arterial/cardiac risk disposition. Anecdotal evidence (the evidence of your own and others' personal experience) has long pointed to this. We all know people who exist on bacon and chip butties but still manage to have 'ideal' blood pressure and cholesterol levels. Yet there are others who are as thin as a rake and never so much as look at a piece of cheese and who die young from heart disease.

What do we make of this apparent contradiction? As always, the key is to apply common sense. If anyone in your family has suffered heart or artery disease or has high blood pressure, then you know you have one risk factor already, so don't add another by eating saturated animal fats. Nor does it make sense to continue eating calorie-dense animal fats if you have a serious or chronic (long-term) overfat problem. This is one extra source of calories you can frankly do without. If, on the other hand, you have never been particularly keen on fatty foods and your overfat problem was never great or is nearly solved, then you shouldn't become paranoid about eating animal fats.

You may still want to opt for the healthiest option of all by substituting animal fats with mono-unsaturated vegetable and nut oils (especially olive oil). Or like me, steer a compromise. I love the taste of really good-quality olive oil, so I use that nearly all the time – try dipping your bread in a dish of olive oil instead of buttering it. But if I'm going to cook a joint for a special occasion I always choose one with plenty of fat because the flavour is so much better – and I confess I don't always trim the fat off before eating! Food is meant to be enjoyed. And if you don't enjoy your eating plan you won't stick to it.

- **Stop**: Lard; dripping; margarine; deep-frying oils.
- **Substitute**: Sparing olive oil; lemon juice/tomato juice/ vinegar for sautéing, moistening and softening in cooking and sauces/dressings.

Condiments

The reasons for stopping the condiments listed below are self-explanatory. In each case it is quite easy to see that they are calorie-dense by virtue of added sugar or added fat. In any case I think we rely far too much on condiments to disguise the poor quality of the food we are eating. When I realised I couldn't stomach a sausage unless it was smothered in tomato ketchup I gave up both the sausage and the ketchup and did myself a favour in the process. Good, fresh food imaginatively prepared

has no need of condiments, as super-chef Marco Pierre White
will tell you with the aid of his meat cleaver.

- **Stop**: Jam; peanut butter; mayonnaise; sandwich spreads;
  commercial dips; salad cream; ready-made cook-in sauces
  and mixes.

- **Substitute**: Honey; Marmite/Bovril; low-cal mayonnaise,
  salad cream, etc.; cottage cheese or yoghurt-based mixes
  for dipping and sandwich spreading; home-made sauces
  based on plain tomato purée (for thick sauces use cornflour
  and skimmed milk or yoghurt, not a butter and flour roux).

Beverages

Alcohol has to be one of the supreme examples of a refined food.
We have taken the innocent grape or wheat ear or humble oat (or
even potato) and turned it into a nutritional devil. Calorie-dense,
almost completely nutrient-free, mildly toxic (poisonous if taken
in excess) – how can we have done such a thing? Because it's jolly
nice, of course, and life would be less fun without it.

I am not a teetotaller, nor am I advocating it, but I think at
least to begin with you have to cut out alcohol altogether on your
low-calorie eating plan. Once you're feeling happily settled and
adjusted to your eating plan you can gradually reintroduce it.
But before every alcoholic drink, always ask yourself: 'Would
something else do?' The more you ask the more likely you are to
discover that a Diet Coke or a mineral water or a cup of coffee
would in fact do equally well, so drink that instead. Sometimes it
won't, so cheers!

- **Stop**: Alcohol; full cream milky and sweetened milky
  drinks; sugary soft drinks, squashes and colas.

- **Substitute**: Mineral water; unsweetened fruit juice; fruit
  flavoured mineral water; tomato juice; diet mixers; diet
  colas; diet soft drinks; skimmed milk or yoghurt shakes.

Eating Out and Take-away

Restaurants and steak houses, even simple cafés and bistros, are now so much more sophisticated that I can't imagine not being able to choose a pleasant, reasonably low-calorie meal when eating out. Really it is just a matter of not kidding yourself. At a steak house, for example, you know perfectly well that melon or soup is lower-calorie than prawn cocktail. It doesn't take a nutritional genius to work out that ordering grilled sole and baked potato for your main course is going to give you fewer calories than steak and chips. So make your decision, but don't kid yourself that you can't eat healthily because you're not eating at home.

Take-away is a different matter. It tends to be ethnic/peasant food. Fish and chips, for example, is British ethnic food; pizza is Italian ethnic food; chicken chow mein is Chinese ethnic food; kebab is Greek ethnic food and so on. Recipes and cooking techniques for ethnic food vary very widely. Even fish and chips can be nutritionally very different depending on whether your meal was fried in lard or vegetable oil.

So when you eat take-away you are taking a nutritional gamble. On the whole Greek take-away is nutritionally best (providing you avoid the taramasalata). A grilled lamb kebab and salad in a pitta bread will not take your eating plan far off course.

Chinese take-away can be high in sugars, oils and additives, but on the compensatory side can be very healthy if you choose the right dishes – nothing deep-fried, not sweet and sour or meat, but mainly vegetable based, and stick to plain boiled rather than fried rice.

Indian take-away can be very fatty, since a clarified butter called ghee is often the base for cooking a dish. Again, common sense will tell you which dishes to order – tikka and tandoor grilled dishes are lower in fat and calories than those with heavy, fatty sauces.

With two-career couples and high pressure lives we tend to rely on take-away increasingly. Don't set yourself impossible goals by trying to do without it altogether, but reach a reasonable compromise by choosing healthier options.

AT-A-GLANCE GUIDE TO STOP AND SUBSTITUTE FOODS

Stop – *Substitute*

Complex Carbohydrate Food Group

white bread – *granary bread*
muesli – *porridge/oat flakes*
flour – *cornflour (for thickening)*

Refined Carbohydrate Food Group

cakes – *soda bread with honey and cottage cheese*
biscuits – *low-cal crispbread with Marmite/Bovril/cottage cheese*
sugar – *honey/low-cal sweetener*
syrup – *fresh fruit juice*
commercial puddings and desserts – *'diet' fromage frais*
sweetened breakfast cereal – *porridge*

pâtisserie – *oatcake topped with fresh fruit and thick low-cal yoghurt*
croissants – *hot granary rolls*
doughnuts – *rice cakes with honey*
alcohol – *mineral water/sparkling fruit juice (no sugar)/diet drinks*

Protein Food Group

sausages – *lean ham/vegetarian sausages*
fried meats and fish – *grilled meats and fish*
pâté – *Marmite/Bovril*
Scotch egg – *plain hard-boiled egg*
pork pie – *ham sandwich*
fatty meat – *lean meat*
peanuts – *potato crisps/olives/cocktail pickles*
taramasalata – *tzatsiki (cucumber blended with yoghurt)*
Chinese take-away – *home-made Chinese (see recipes, p. 325)*
Indian take-away – *Greek take-away*

Vegetable and Fruit Food Group

chips – *stir-fried carrot and parsnip sticks*

roast potatoes – *baked or mashed potatoes*

deep-fried onion rings – *sautéed onion*

sweetened fruit juice – *fresh squeezed orange juice*

Dairy Food Group

full cream milk – *skimmed milk*

cream – *yoghurt/fromage frais*

cream cheese – *cottage cheese*

chocolates – *banana/Ryvita sandwich*

milk shakes – *yoghurt shakes*

Fats Group

butter – *low fat spread*

fats – *olive oil*

frying oils – *lemon juice/tomato juice/vinegar*

Condiments

jam – *honey*

peanut butter – *Marmite/Bovril*

mayonnaise – *low-cal salad cream*

sandwich spreads – *Marmite/Bovril/cottage cheese*

commercial dips – *home-made yoghurt dips*

Beverages

alcohol – *diet beverages/Virgin Mary, etc.*

sweetened drinks – *unsweetened and diet drinks*

malted/milky drinks – *skimmed milk/yoghurt drinks*

SAMPLE SUBSTITUTION PROGRAMME

* Items marked with an asterisk are given in greater detail in the Snack Substitutes and Recipes sections (pp. 313, 324).

MONDAY

Breakfast

Normal 2 slices white toast with butter and jam; sugar frosted cereal with full cream milk; sweetened orange juice; coffee with milk and sugar

Includes these Stop Foods White bread, butter, jam, sugary cereal, full cream milk, sweetened orange juice, sugar

Substitute 2 slices granary bread toast with low-fat spread and Marmite; *pure oat flakes with skimmed milk; fresh squeezed orange juice; coffee with skimmed milk, no sugar

Elevenses

Normal 1 doughnut; coffee with skimmed milk and sugar

Stop Doughnut, sugar

Substitute *1 plain oatcake; coffee with skimmed milk

Lunch

Normal Chips; sausage roll and peas; apple tart; 1 glass wine

Stop Chips, sausage roll, apple tart, wine

Substitute Large bowl of soup; ham and salad; apple; sparkling mineral water

Afternoon tea

Normal Piece of cake; cup of tea without sugar

Stop Cake

Substitute 2 slices brown bread spread with honey and cottage cheese; cup of tea with skimmed milk

Dinner

Normal Prawn cocktail with 2 slices brown bread and butter; pasta in home-made tomato sauce with courgettes; ice-cream

Stop Butter, ice-cream

Substitute Prawn cocktail with 2 slices brown bread spread with low-fat spread; *pasta in home-made tomato sauce with courgettes; *plain yoghurt mashed with frozen raspberries

TUESDAY

Breakfast

Normal 1 soft-boiled egg with 2 slices bread and butter; fresh orange juice; black coffee

Stop Butter
Substitute I soft-boiled egg with 2 slices bread and low-fat spread; fresh orange juice; black coffee

Elevenses

Normal American-style cookie; coffee with milk and sugar
Stop Cookie, whole milk, sugar
Substitute Orange; coffee with skimmed milk, no sugar

Lunch

Normal Fried chicken limb in breadcrumbs; chips; peas; individual portion fruit trifle; glass wine; coffee with milk and sugar
Stop Fried meat, chips, trifle, wine, coffee with milk and sugar
Substitute Grilled chicken limb (remove skin); mashed potato; peas; fruit salad with yoghurt; sparkling mineral water; black coffee

Afternoon tea

Normal Small bar of chocolate; tea with skimmed milk
Stop Chocolate
Substitute *Banana and Ryvita sandwich

Dinner

Normal Packet of peanuts; sausages; baked beans; 2 slices buttered toast; flavoured jelly; 2 glasses wine; black coffee; I chocolate truffle
Stop Peanuts, sausages, butter, wine, truffle
Substitute Packet of potato crisps; 2 egg Spanish omelette made with skimmed milk; baked beans; 2 slices toast with low-fat spread; *portion plain creamy yoghurt sprinkled with honey and walnuts; *Piermont; black coffee; tangerine

WEDNESDAY

Breakfast

Normal Sugary cereal with milk; 2 chocolate biscuits; fresh squeezed orange juice; black coffee
Stop Sugary cereal, whole milk, chocolate biscuits

Substitute Oatflakes with skimmed milk and chopped banana; 2 Ryvitas with low-fat spread and Marmite; fresh squeezed orange juice; coffee

Elevenses

Normal Shortcake biscuit; coffee with milk and sugar
Stop Shortcake biscuit, whole milk, sugar
Substitute *Rice cake spread with flavoured cottage cheese; coffee with skimmed milk, no sugar

Lunch

Normal Scotch egg salad; 2 slices brown bread and butter; apple; wine; coffee
Stop Scotch egg, butter, wine
Substitute 2 slices smoked ham; large continental salad; 2 slices bread with low-fat spread; mineral water; coffee

Afternoon tea

Normal Snack bar; tea with skimmed milk, no sugar
Stop Snack bar
Substitute *Oatcake; tea

Dinner

Normal Bowl of soup; grilled lamb chop; spinach; mashed potato; tinned tomato; fresh unsugared fruit salad; coffee with skimmed milk, no sugar
Stop None
Substitute None

THURSDAY

Breakfast

Normal 2 rashers of bacon and 1 fried egg on buttered toast; fresh orange juice; black coffee
Stop Fried bacon, fried egg, butter

Substitute 2 rashers of well-grilled bacon and 2 whole grilled tomatoes on toast with low-fat spread; fresh orange juice; black coffee

Elevenses

Normal Chocolate digestive biscuit; hot chocolate drink

Stop Biscuit, hot chocolate

Substitute *2 Ryvitas spread with honey and flavoured cottage cheese; *warm skimmed milk with 2 or 3 drops vanilla essence

Lunch

Normal Baked potato with cream cheese and chives; salad with mayonnaise; chocolate gâteau; black coffee; Coca Cola

Stop Cream cheese, mayonnaise, chocolate gâteau, Coca Cola

Substitute Baked potato with grated cheese or cottage cheese; salad with *vinegar and lemon juice dressing or low-cal salad cream; *mashed banana with yoghurt and crumbled oatcake; coffee; Diet Coke

Afternoon tea

Normal Egg sandwich; tea

Stop Butter, mayonnaise

Substitute Sandwich of sliced egg and tomato on brown, hold the mayo, hold the butter; tea

Dinner

Normal Taramasalata with brown bread and butter; commercially prepared cod and salmon fish pie; spinach; grilled tomatoes; ice-cream; 2 glasses wine; coffee; after-dinner mint

Stop Taramasalata, ice-cream, wine, mint

Substitute *Tzatsiki with water biscuits; check label on fish pie and substitute *home-made if it contains more than 30 per cent fat; *frozen yoghurt; *Piermont; black coffee; 2 dates

FRIDAY

Breakfast

Normal Toast with butter and jam; milky coffee

Stop Butter, jam, whole milk

Substitute 2 slices toast with low-fat spread and Marmite; coffee made with hot skimmed milk; fresh orange juice

Elevenses

Normal Apple; coffee with skimmed milk

Stop None

Substitute None

Lunch

Normal Pork pie with chutney; tomato salad; 2 glasses wine; black coffee

Stop Pork pie, wine

Substitute Beef sandwich (no butter); tomato salad; fresh orange juice; coffee

Afternoon tea

Normal Ginger biscuit; tea

Stop Ginger biscuit

Substitute *Ryvita and flavoured cottage cheese; tea

Dinner

Normal 3 measures spirit; Chinese take-away; 2 glasses wine; milky coffee; mint

Stop Alcohol, Chinese take-away, milky coffee, mint

Substitute Diet Coke; *home-made Chinese; China tea (no milk); orange quarters

SATURDAY

Breakfast

Normal 1 slice buttered toast; black coffee

Stop Butter

Substitute Toast with low-fat spread; coffee; sparkling mineral water

Elevenses

Normal Doughnut; coffee

Stop Doughnut

Substitute Egg custard tart; coffee. While not very low-calorie, at least the egg custard is less fatty and sugary than a doughnut and you should be allowed a compromise at weekends!

Lunch

Normal Pub lunch of bread, butter, cheese, chutney, salad, chips; ½ pint shandy

Stop Butter, chips, shandy

Substitute Pub lunch of bread, cheese, no butter, extra salad, one pack potato crisps; tomato juice or Diet Coke

Afternoon tea

Normal Cake; tea

Stop Cake

Substitute Honey and cottage cheese on Ryvita; tea

Dinner

Normal 2 measures spirit; avocado filled with prawns; fried steak; peas; baked potato; grilled tomatoes and mushrooms; ice-cream; 3 glasses wine

Stop Alcohol, fried steak, ice-cream

Substitute Diet drink; avocado filled with prawns; well-grilled steak; peas; baked potato; grilled tomatoes and mushrooms; fresh fruit salad; sparkling mineral water

SUNDAY

Breakfast

Normal Fried bacon; sausage; fried bread; grilled tomatoes; orange juice; coffee

Stop Fried bacon, sausage, fried bread

Substitute Well-grilled bacon; poached egg on toast; grilled tomatoes; fresh squeezed orange juice; coffee

No elevenses today

Lunch
Normal 2 measures spirit; roast pork; mashed potato; cabbage; peas; gravy; apple pie with cream; black coffee

Stop Alcohol, roast meat, apple pie, cream

Substitute Mineral water/tomato juice; *low-fat pork casserole; mashed potato; cabbage; peas; gravy; *stewed fruit (oranges, bananas, peeled sliced apples) with yoghurt and a garnish of crumbled oatcake; coffee

Afternoon tea
Normal Biscuit; tea

Stop Biscuit

Substitute I slice toasted soda bread with honey; tea

Dinner
Normal Mushroom omelette; salad; bread with low-fat spread; cheese; celery; 2 glasses wine

Stop Wine

Substitute Mushroom omelette; salad; bread; cheese; celery; *Piermont

---

VARIATION: THE LOW-CALORIE EATING PLAN FOR THE CONGENITALLY OBESE

Have you had an overfat problem for as long as you can remember? Were you a big baby? Are your parents overfat?

Doctors now recognise that many of those with chronic overfat problems are in fact congenitally obese. That means they have been fat from birth. Unfortunately the prognosis (outlook) for those who are congenitally obese is not good.

It is much harder for the congenitally obese to lose fat and maintain the loss. Those who were slim as children and teenagers but gained fat in adulthood have every chance of losing that fat fairly quickly and maintaining the loss, providing they improve their eating habits and to some extent their lifestyle. The same is not true for the congenitally obese, and, despite considerable research, scientists are still not quite sure why this should be. Various theories have been put forward. Some believe the congenitally obese have fewer brown fat cells, which means they may have less capacity to activate and burn up fat reserves. Others think that the main reason is environmental. Poor parental eating habits, and possibly being fed cow's milk rather than breast milk, are cited as possible causes. One widely quoted myth is that the congenitally obese have a slower metabolism than the naturally slim. In fact the opposite is true. Congenitally obese people tend to be heavier than slim people and this means their metabolism actually has to work harder to support and sustain body weight.

Statistical surveys have revealed that there is some sort of genetic link between parental overfat and congenital obesity. The equation works out as follows:

Two obese parents = 70 per cent likelihood of congenital obesity

One obese parent = 40 per cent likelihood of congenital obesity

Nil obese parents = 10 per cent likelihood of congenital obesity

Researchers know that this link must be mainly genetic because of studies of twins brought up in different households. Looking at twins born to obese parents and separated at birth, they discovered that even where one twin was raised by lean foster parents that twin was still just as likely to be overfat as its sibling raised by obese parents.

The child raised by obese parents also faces the additional problem that it is likely to pick up poor eating habits which must be unlearnt in later life.

As the child of two lean parents myself, it seems to me desperately unfair that nature has loaded the dice in this way against some people. It also seems to be an almost impossible trap to escape.

The commercial slimming industry doesn't help. Pushing so-called slimming products at people who have a chronic problem seems immoral to me. It is also sad that the congenitally obese are constantly presented with images of the human body which they have little or no chance of attaining themselves. Repeated yo-yo slimming attempts only make the situation worse, because persistent conventional slimming diets eventually lower the metabolism by up to 10 per cent, making things even more difficult for the congenitally obese.

So if you've been fat for as long as you can remember, I'm afraid the outlook is bleak. There are no two ways about it. You are going to find it tough to get slim.

There you are. That's the truth all those miracle slimming products never tell you. It is going to be difficult. Worse still, you may not succeed. In fact I have to tell you now that you almost certainly won't succeed 100 per cent.

No, don't stop reading. I'm not promising you complete success but I can show you how not to fail completely. Look at the percentages. Isn't it better to try to get half-way there and make it, rather than try to get the whole way and fall flat on your face before you've gone a yard? Wouldn't it be nicer to be permanently and successfully a bit slimmer than forever pursuing the unattainable goal of being thin?

This is the big mistake most congenitally overfat slimmers make. They try to reach a goal weight that is genetically impossible for them to attain, much less sustain. They're conned into believing it is both possible and necessary for them to do this when in fact it is neither.

Here's some good news: being above ideal weight is not a health risk in itself. Only those who are seriously above ideal weight for a prolonged period of time actually jeopardise their health. The statistics show that amid all the hype over slimming, very few people know these facts. Look at the figures (for 1991, from the Department of Health report *The Health of the Nation*, published 1994):

- **Group A** – 58 per cent of women and 49 per cent of men in England are around (or below) ideal weight.
- **Group B** – 26 per cent of women and 39 per cent of men in England are overweight, although not to the extent of being a serious threat to their health.
- **Group C** – 16 per cent of women and 12 per cent of men in England are obese to the point of threatening health
- NOTE – 75 per cent of people in Britain go on slimming diets (90 per cent of women).

Any way you add it up, that means that more than a third of the people who go on conventional slimming diets don't need to. And more than a half of the people who slim don't need to do it for the sake of their health.

Now let's look at these figures from the point of view of the congenitally obese. At the moment you are likely to be among the approximately 30 per cent (group B), possibly even the 15 per cent (group C), and in a perfect world you would like to be among the 50 per cent of people (group A) who are around ideal weight.

This may not be possible. What is much more achievable is to step out of the 15 per cent group and into the 30 per cent group, going from group C to group B; or if your problem is less severe you could go from group B to the top end of the ideal group A.

This is the heart of the plan for the congenitally obese. It is the art of success through compromise. Our aim is the achievable. I hope that the incentive of real hope of some degree of success will help you get through this tough task.

Now let's get started. Follow the plan step by step. You'll be using the same eating plan as the low-calorie planner, but your approach will be different.

STEP 1: HOW OBESE ARE YOU?

The diagram (on p.58) is derived from Quetelet's Index, a method originally devised by a Belgian scientist to show degrees of obesity, now widely accepted. The graph shows five areas of height/weight ratio, as follows:

–A This group is below ideal weight.
A This group is at ideal weight.
B Heavy end of the Department of Health 'desirable' weight statistics, that is definitely over ideal weight but not so much so as to be out of the average reasonable weight range.
C Clinically obese (seriously overweight).
D Dangerously obese (severe health risk).

If you are in group D your aim is to get to group C. If you are in group C your aim is to get to group B.

● NOTE: If you are already in group B and have remained in that group for pretty much all your life, regardless of slimming attempts, then it is very likely that you are in fact at the correct weight for you as an individual. This eating plan is unlikely to be helpful to you. I recommend you accept your group B weight. If you are unwilling to do that you could consider looking at the

THE OBESITY INDEX

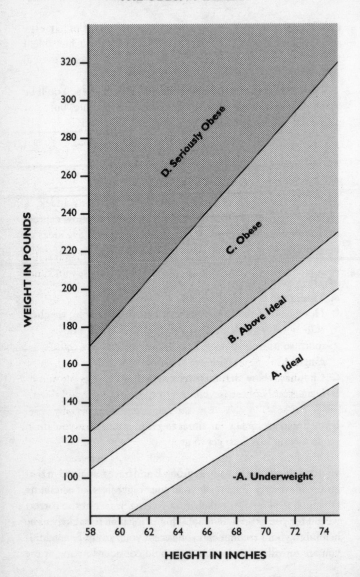

Low-allergen eating plan, which is often successful in cases of chronic obesity.

STEP 2: LOW-CALORIE EATING PLAN

Turn back to the Low-calorie Eating Plan (p. 27) and read it thoroughly. Start the plan and follow it just as if you had a normal overfat problem. But you will also need some extra help. The next step, mind tricks, is designed to help counteract the effects of being congenitally obese.

STEP 3: MIND TRICKS

If you are congenitally obese the Low-calorie Eating Plan is right for you nutritionally, but you should also follow these mind and body tricks.

I. Appetite Control

● **Always drink before eating**
Research has shown that many congenitally obese people find it hard to distinguish between the sensations of hunger and thirst. This is not actually very surprising, since eating (especially very sweet or tasty foods) has the effect of making saliva flow and thus moistening the mouth.

Next time you feel peckish especially if it is between meals, drink a glass of liquid (preferably mineral water or fresh squeezed juice) and then see of you still feel the need for something to eat.

Also get into the habit of having a glass of water or juice before you start your meal. You will find it will kill your appetite slightly and you will feel full sooner.

● **Control portion size**

Seconds, thirds and fourths are often the downfall of the long-term overfat rather than the actual food being eaten. Congenitally obese people do seem to be able to eat more at a sitting than naturally slim people. Very often also there is a deep-rooted aversion to leaving food uneaten on the table. Overcome this by never putting the serving dish on the dining table. Serve yourself a plate full of food in the kitchen and then take the plate to the table. This will not necessarily stop you from eating seconds, but it will make it a conscious decision rather than a reflex action.

When eating alone, never cook more than one portion's worth. Don't kid yourself you will save left-overs for another time.

Never serve nibbly foods (biscuits, cheese, nuts, etc.) straight out of the pack. Take out a serving, put it on a separate dish, put the rest of the food back in the cupboard or fridge and then take the plate of nibbles away to where you plan to eat them.

Never keep food, especially chocolates and sweets, anywhere in the house except the kitchen or larder.

If you want to have a snack in front of the television, don't grab the packet and sit down with it. In the kitchen prepare a reasonable sized snack; serve it on to a plate; put the rest of the ingredients away before carrying the plate through to the television.

If all this seems like far too much trouble then you are obviously not really hungry – makes you think doesn't it?

● **Substitute bulk**

Since birth human beings have the desire to put things into their mouths. It begins with the nipple and goes on through comfort rags, thumb-sucking, sweet-eating, nail-biting, gum-chewing and smoking. For many people putting food into their mouths fulfils this basic need, but unfortunately the general reflex is to chew and swallow this food. (Interestingly, bulimics tend to have overcome this reflex and will regurgitate and spit out food at will (see the section on Eating Disorders, p. 120).

If you are a seeker after 'oral comfort' as it is clinically defined, you will find it very hard to overcome the basic need to put something into your mouth – especially when you are concentrating on something. Using a comfort rag is obviously one option, but not something most adults would care to be seen doing. Instead, make sure that the food you use for oral comfort is not calorie-dense and ideally takes a long time to eat. Here are some suggestion:

Raw Brussels sprouts
Raw carrot sticks
Olives (use sparingly)
Sprouted beans (from your supermarket) sprinkled with seasoning and lemon juice
Chopped apples
Dates
Dried figs
Fresh fruit (especially cherries, grapes and strawberries)
Dry crispbreads
All Bran
Plain popcorn
Wholegrains (remember the yokel chewing his straw?)
Raw peas (defrosted frozen peas are fairly sweet)

In times of famine and drought, humans have assuaged their need for oral comfort by putting inedible objects like small pebbles and pieces of leather or string in their mouths. These could be sucked and chewed, giving the illusion of eating and tricking the mind into feeling less hungry. It is a terrible irony that in these times of plenty we are using precisely the same technique to trick ourselves out of eating the readily available food which surrounds us.

● **Be an Active Eater**

People who have been overfat for a long time tend not to have a very mature or discerning approach to food – whether this is a cause or an effect of overfatness is hard to tell.

One famous experiment compared the reactions of two groups of people left in a waiting-room with food available. In the first part of the experiment the food was two bowls of peanuts, one shelled and the other unshelled. The first group, fat people, ate the shell-off nuts first, moving on to the shell-on nuts only when the other nuts were finished and they were still being kept waiting. The second group, slim people, browsed equally among the shelled and unshelled nuts and tended to stop eating at a certain point, no matter how long they were left waiting.

In the second part of the experiment the groups were left in the waiting-room with only a bowl of shell-on peanuts. The researchers were surprised to discover that the fat people tended not even to begin eating the shell-on peanuts, whereas the slim people ate roughly the same amount of nuts as they had before.

This suggested several interesting theories. The most obvious was that the fat people were lazy eaters compared with the slim people – they ate all the food that was readily accessible but very little of the food that required some form of preparation. Also the fat people tended to be passive, unconscious eaters. If it was easy for them to begin eating they would do so, and once started they would continue to eat almost as a reflex, even if it became more difficult.

By contrast the slim people were much more actively engaged in the eating process. They made conscious decisions about eating, chose to eat a more difficult but more rewarding food, and were able to stop eating at some point.

Passive eating seems to be a major problem for congenitally obese people. It is often said that thin people have to remember to eat; fat people have to remember not to eat. So try to develop food consciousness and turn yourself from a passive to an active eater. That means thinking about the food you are eating before, during and after eating. Try these techniques:

- If you fancy a snack, decide: 'You can eat anything you want, but it must be the thing you *most* want. If you can't get hold of the thing you *most* want or you don't know what it is, then you can't have something to eat.'
- Eat meals that take a lot of preparation. Enjoy the preparation. Present the food attractively, even if you are eating alone.
- When you are eating, put your knife and fork down between mouthfuls. If you are eating with someone, start an interesting conversation.
- Decide what order you are going to eat foods on your plate and why. After each mouthful, mentally analyse how it tasted and whether it was satisfying.
- At the end of a meal, think about the food you have eaten and decide whether and why you liked it. Admit to yourself if you didn't like it.
- Never eat the first thing you lay your hands on.

2. Exercise

- **Begin exercise**

This is not an exercise book. Despite what many people think, exercise alone very rarely results in fat loss. However, exercise is a great ally for the congenitally obese, largely because beginning a programme of exercise represents one important thing: a **change** in the existing situation. In a passive, unsatisfactory situation like chronic overfat, anything which **changes** the long-standing circumstances is an important step forward, even if it doesn't immediately lead to achieving the goal.

Exercise may change many things about you. If you do enough it may increase your calorie requirements. If you do not eat more this will have the same effect as reducing your calorie intake. In my experience, however, most people do eat more when they start exercising, so don't rely on this too much.

Exercise can also counteract the metabolism-lowering effect of dieting. If you take it fairly gently and keep at it regularly, exercise can improve your health and fitness (though again this has often been overrated).

Perhaps the most important benefit of exercise, though, is that it is physical. In order to exercise at all, the overfat person has to start thinking about their body. Lack of body awareness is one of the roots of chronic overfatness. Someone who is not in tune with their body doesn't treat it very well. They may even come to dislike it and then want to punish it. Doing something physical forces you to get in touch with your body again, to listen to it and recognise its importance to you. The well-being generated by physical activity can also lead to you learning to like your body.

In my view this achievement of regaining contact with your body and faith in it does more to combat overfat than any other single factor.

• Get outdoors

Exercise taken outdoors tends to be more effective in stress reduction and improvement in self-esteem. Try taking a walk in your local park or the countryside whenever you can. This has the added advantage that it keeps you away from food for longer. Exercise in a sports centre tends to be followed by a binge in the centre's cafeteria.

• Exercise before eating

Not only is this recommended from the point of view of digestion and safety, but there is also some evidence to suggest that appetite may be reduced after exercise which raises the temperature of the body. Personally I'm normally ravenous after exercise, but there may be something in it.

3. Lifestyle

● **Keep your hands busy**

As we have noted, one of the chronically overfat person's main problems is passive eating. The hand that unconsciously reaches out for another crisp or another piece of chocolate is your worst enemy. We have to do anything and everything we can to combat that.

One of the simplest ways of all is both logical and utterly basic: if you already have your hands full, you can't pick up something to eat. Yes, of course you can put down whatever is in your hands so that you can then pick up something to eat. But it's an extra step. Only a little one, maybe, but it's enough to make the act of eating something a conscious one, to turn you from a passive to an active eater. You'll be amazed how much less you graze and nibble if your hands are already occupied. Here are some hands-on activities you could try:

Needlework (darning, mending)
Knitting
Ten-finger typing
Tapestry/rug making
Drawing/painting
Crosswords/puzzles
Fly-tying
Hand-held computer games
Woodwork/carving/carpentry

● **Beware television**

If we are honest with ourselves, television is a pretty boring form of entertainment. When was the last time you watched the television and were so riveted that nobody spoke; nobody got up to switch the lights on; nobody made a cup of tea; nobody read a magazine; nobody passed the chocolates round; nobody even fell asleep? Isn't the picture when we're watching television more likely to be one of people coming in and out; bringing food; doing tasks; reading the paper; chatting; dozing off?

The trouble with television is that it isn't absorbing enough on its own. Unless you're completely exhausted you really need to be doing something else while you're watching. Like eating.

To begin with I suggest you make a **change** in your normal situation by giving up television watching for a while and doing something else. Maybe your television time could turn into your exercise period. When you're beginning to get slimmer by all means start watching again, but keep your hands busy while you are doing it.

● **Plan your life/career goals**

In researching this section of the book I spoke to many people who had been overfat right through childhood and into early adulthood. Slim now, most of them said they had lost their excess fat *for no apparent reason*. Most strenuously denied having consciously dieted. In fact, one young woman said: 'I actually gave up dieting, I just didn't have the time to diet.'

This put me on to the track. Without exception the people who had lost fat for no apparent reason had all been through a change in lifestyle. One had moved house; another had gone to university. The girl who didn't have time to diet had been promoted into a challenging new job.

Almost certainly all of them were in fact eating less than they had before, but because they were so preoccupied with their change in circumstances they hadn't noticed it. In fact they had been so absorbed by their new lives that they hadn't had time to think about food much at all.

An externally imposed change in circumstances had given all these people the opportunity to put eating and food into perspective.

The chronically overfat often put their eating problems at the top of their concerns, leaving other far more important elements like career, marriage and family neglected. I advise you to make a conscious effort to put the genuinely important things in life at the forefront of your thinking. Assess your present situation and work out how you might like to change it. You could try for a different job; aim for promotion; renew your relationship with your spouse; make more time for your children.

Being overfat is not the most important thing in your life. Find out what is and concentrate on it, and you may just find overfat ceases to be a problem.

● **Pursue new interests**
As I have stressed, **change** is the most important ally in a campaign against chronic overfat. You may not feel up to tackling the big things – career, marriage, family – at the beginning, but almost any change will be for the better.

Start small. Join the local photographic society. Begin compiling a history of your family as far back as you can go. Learn how to swim. Take the advanced motoring test. Anything will do so long as it's different.

4. Emotions

● **Be positive**
It is all too easy to let chronic overfat alter your outlook on life. With today's fashion for slimness particularly there is a sense of failure attached to being overfat. It is important to remind yourself that there are far more serious things in life than whether you are fat or slim – like being alive for example. Remember that only a tiny percentage of people are overfat to such a degree as to be a serious danger to their life (incidentally, it is roughly the same proportion as those for whom being too thin is a threat).

So if it's not actually threatening your life you can get on with living, can't you? Be positive about your life – don't waste a moment more of it than you need to on your overfat problem.

● **Reward yourself**

It's very important to congratulate yourself each time you make a little headway. First of all give yourself credit for the strides you are making, whether it is in fat loss or in other ways, like taking up new interests or taking exercise. Remember, though, that food should no longer have the central importance in your life, so try not to use it as a reward. There are lots of other ways you can reward yourself. A few are listed below, and you'll be able to think of others:

● Take a day off work.
● Arrange an outing with spouse or friends.
● Have an evening with a favourite video.
● Go to a football match/any sport you enjoy watching.
● Have a weekend away.
● Have a beauty treatment.
● Buy some magazines and plan a make-over.
● Go shopping.
● Treat yourself to a new gadget/accessory you've been wanting for some time.
● Take a long luxurious bath.

● **Consider counselling**

Many therapists and nutritionists working with the chronically overfat are discovering that there are often psychological and emotional reasons why someone has difficulty losing fat. Among the case histories I have seen are those of a woman who had been abused as a child and gradually developed her layers of fat as a physical protection. Without her fat she discovered she would have felt very vulnerable. Therapy (including hypnotherapy) enabled her to come to terms with the childhood abuse and she was eventually able to lose some of her overfat.

In another case a young man had constantly been pushed by his parents, who were highly authoritarian. Although he became a high achiever he also gained a great deal of excess fat. During the course of psychotherapy he mentioned that he had never felt comfortable with or accepting of his body. Working with his therapist, he discovered that he had projected his parents' disapproval of his personality on to his own body. He had been brought up to feel that he was deserving of disapproval, but as he achieved more in his career, the only way he was able to enact that disapproval was by developing a body that failed to meet today's standards of physical success. Gradually he freed himself of the impact of that early parental disapproval and at the same time lost some (though not all) of his overfat.

It may be that your overfat problem has an emotional or psychological root. If you would like to explore this there are lots of ways of getting in touch with counsellors, therapists and psychiatric practitioners (all slightly different disciplines). Discuss it with your family doctor or check the addresses on p. 334.

• Learn self-acceptance

It is extraordinary what a battleground the body has become today. Overeaters; undereaters; compulsive exercisers; couch potatoes; cosmetic surgery addicts; self-mutilators – all are punishing themselves by being unkind to their bodies.

People with a genuine physical disability must wonder at our inability to recognise what a fantastic piece of machinery we have been given in our body. It doesn't really matter what a healthy adult body looks like on the outside, the fact is that it has the most amazing powers. It can give you an orgasm. It enables you to smell the lilac or admire a sunset. The skin is waterproof so that you can go swimming without sinking. The legs are strong enough to carry your whole weight, so you can stand upright and leave your hands free to do all sorts of interesting things.

Best of all, your body contains the organs that stimulate and nourish the brain and heart. So your body is extremely important. If you are feeling unhappy, guilty or anxious about something, don't take it out on your body. Ultimately it won't make you feel any better and you could end up even worse off – without a body that works well, for example.

So many of us have things we punish ourselves for, and how do we stop? Learning self-acceptance is a good start. It would take a whole book fully to discuss what self-acceptance is, but here are a few keys:

- Value yourself and recognise your talents.
- Give yourself permission to be yourself.
- Allow yourself to be tired or lazy when the need arises.
- Notice your flaws and try to improve, but also forgive yourself for them.

5. Diet Products

• 'Light' products

Used carefully, 'diet', 'low-cal' and 'light' foods can be a great help in fighting chronic overfatness. But as with all commercially manufactured food products, it is vital to read the label carefully and understand fully the claims being made.

A 'diet' product should have significantly fewer calories than the ordinary version of it. So Diet Coke has only one calorie per can, far fewer than original Coca Cola.

'Low-cal' will be comparatively low in calories – but many foods are beginning to be labelled this way when they are naturally low in calories anyway, which can be confusing.

'Light' products are even more confusing. Originating in America, this title is applied to all sorts of foods which are not low in calories at all. 'Lite' beer, for example, is simply brewed in a slightly different way.

Read the notes on Food Labelling on p. 14, and once you feel sure what foods really are lower in calories there is no reason not to incorporate them into your day-to-day eating.

● **Meal replacements**

Nutritionists universally condemn these products, which consist of a sweet chocolate biscuit or snack bar, or a sweet shake drink which is used to replace one or two meals a day.

The primary problem with these products is that they do nothing to break bad eating habits. Chocolates, snacks and shakes will *never* be the basis for sound nutrition, no matter what claims are made for them.

Nor are these meal replacements particularly low in calories. The average meal replacement is about 200 or 300 calories, and yet when you have eaten one all you have done is eat a snack bar or drink a shake. If you are a clever low-calorie eating planner you can easily rustle yourself up a satisfying and nutritious meal for the same amount of calories. You could have a plain one-egg omelette, a massive salad and a slice of bread for the same calories.

You could of course also have an ordinary snack bar or milk shake plus a multivitamin pill and a bran tablet, and you would have the same nutritional value and the same number of calories as a meal replacement.

Very few low-calorie dieters I know would plan to eat more than 300 calories each for breakfast and lunch, so what is the point of buying meal replacements?

6. Stabilising

● **Be realistic in your goals**

It is far more helpful to set a realistic goal and achieve it than to set an impossible goal and fail. Most congenitally obese people were never intended by nature to be truly skinny and you'll just have to accept it. This doesn't mean you have to be massively overfat, but it does mean that if you ever do get down to a very thin measurement you may well rebound into increased overfatness. So try to aim for a body shape that you can stick at for long periods of time.

Many women find that the weight and body shape they stabilised at between puberty and the end of adolescence is the realistic one for them to attain (this is less true of men for biological reasons). If you were naturally fairly slim for most of the years between 12 and 18 you have a very good chance of becoming so again. If you were consistently overfat or were a yo-yo dieter at that period it is going to be much more difficult for you to find the right weight at which to stabilise.

● Aim not to gain

Once you have reached a sensible degree of fatness it is very important to stabilise. That means not gaining fat – but equally importantly, it also means not losing more. If you go on trying to lose fat you will have defeated the object of the eating plan, because food will still be dominating your life. As long as food is such a major factor in your life you will always be at risk of overeating.

During your stabilisation period the best approach is simply aiming not to gain. The best way to check is to take your measurements and make sure they don't increase. After a long stable period you will be able to tell just from the way your clothes fit. Try not to do it by weighing yourself, as this can become obsessive, and is not a particularly reliable measure. Be logical. You want to look slim, not display a label reading 8 stone 4 pounds 12 ounces.

WHAT NEXT?

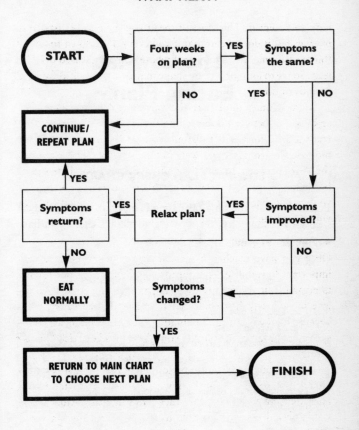

2. The Low-fat Eating Plan

LOW-FAT PLAN CHECK CHART

Before you start the Low-fat Eating Plan, fill in the check chart below by ticking any Yes answers to double-check you have chosen the most appropriate eating plan.

1. Wearing trousers is a problem. ☐
2. I take a larger size in skirts (trousers if male) than jackets. ☐
3. My thighs are my worst figure problem. ☐
4. I don't like any part of my body. ☐
5. I have a very sedentary job. ☐
6. I get very swollen up around waist and hips. ☐
7. I can pinch rolls of fat round hips, buttocks and thighs. ☐
8. I'm always too tired to bother about my figure. ☐
9. I very often eat out or buy take-away food. ☐
10. I love fried food. ☐

Ticks KEY

0–3 A low-fat diet is not the best choice for you. Try to be more specific about your symptoms. For example, if you answered Yes to 4, you may well be a borderline eating disorder candidate, so have a look at the Low-sugar Eating Plan (p. 97).

4–8 Your symptoms suggest you suffer from the commonest problem among the British, especially women – pear-shapedness. The Low-fat Eating Plan is ideal for you.

9–10 So many Yes answers suggest you may have more pressing problems

than your pear-shape. If you answered Yes to 6 or 8, you should
check the Anti-candida and Low-allergen Eating Plans (pp. 228, 259)
before making your choice. If you answered Yes to 9, spend at least
4 weeks on the Low-processing Eating Plan (p. 152) before trying the
Low-fat Eating Plan.

WELCOME TO THE LOW-FAT EATING PLAN

The first thing to do on this eating plan is reassure yourself: you
are not alone! Pear-shapedness is the commonest figure problem
of all among British women (though if you are a pear-shaped
man you are a little out of the ordinary). According to leading
clothes manufacturers, British bottoms are even getting bigger –
so compared with some, yours may actually be quite small! One
mail order company did a huge size survey so that they could be
sure their sizes would fit. They discovered that the woman who
regards herself as size 12 today is in fact more like what a size 14
or even 16 would have been in the late 1940s and the 1950s.

Looking at Kate Moss and all the other super-waif models of
today, you could be forgiven for thinking that plump bottoms
and curvy thighs have disappeared. In fact, it's quite the reverse.
It is far more normal to be big between the knees and waist than
to go straight up and down.

Before we start to whittle them away, let's just appreciate our
bottoms and thighs for a moment. First of all, they are what
anthropologists call a 'secondary sexual characteristic'. That
means that they are one of the ways of telling women from men –
not the most obvious way, but a good one nevertheless. As you
might imagine, this also means that they are one of the factors
that attract men to women. Curving thighs and a pronounced
bottom are very much part of the ideal sexual stereotype of a
woman. If you look at any comic book drawings of female super-

heroines you will notice that they are all drawn (by men) with the sort of thighs you might well prefer not to reveal in a Superwoman outfit.

Apart from its essential femininity, there is a great deal of evidence to show that a larger lower half is also healthier than a larger top half. Studies of heart disease show that those who carry their excess fat below the waist are less likely to get heart disease than those whose excess fat is above the waist, round the upper abdomen and stomach. Since men tend to carry their excess fat around the stomach (beer gut), this may be one of the reasons why men up to the age of 50 are more prone to heart disease than women the same age.

So your particular overfat problem is not as serious as some. Having said that, you are overfat and you obviously want to do something about it. Going on the Low-fat Eating Plan is a good idea for many reasons. Government bodies and nutritionists are currently campaigning for people to eat less fat in their diet whether they are overfat or not.

Several dangers are now associated with too much fat in the diet. The major one which you will have heard a lot about is heart disease. The weight of medical evidence is gathering to support the view that too much saturated – animal – fat in the diet contributes to a raised blood cholesterol level and to arteriosclerosis. Another recent study has pointed to a high-fat diet as a contributing factor in breast cancer. Practitioners of complementary medicine also believe that too much saturated fat promotes the action of biological oxidation, which contributes to ageing.

So there are lots of good reasons for going on the Low-fat Eating Plan. But with your symptoms you will be particularly interested in the idea that the Low-fat Eating Plan will help you to lose fat, especially from your buttocks, hips and thighs.

The idea that a particular eating plan can lead you to lose fat from one area rather than another is quite controversial. Many nutritionists and almost all doctors disregard it altogether. Yet the anecdotal (observed by experience) evidence keeps coming along that women who have reduced the amount of fat in their eating, for whatever reason, have encountered as a side-effect inch loss from their bottoms and thighs.

Doctors will argue that this is purely because a decreased amount of calories is being taken in, due to the reduced amount of fat. But this does not explain why women who go on ordinary general calorie-reduced diets tend not to experience a specific below-the-waist inch loss. If it was due to reduced calories alone, surely any diet should produce the effect? As we all know, this is far from the case. Any woman who has dieted successfully is familiar with the vanishing breast syndrome while the thighs remain as stubbornly jodhpur-shaped as ever.

Without having done any controlled experiments I cannot put forward a supportable theory. My suspicion is that the phenomenon is due to the way fats and sugars are metabolised differently in the body. Sugars are rapidly metabolised and provide instant energy. Energy from sugars is the first to be called upon by the body to provide fuel for day-to-day life. Spare fuel is stored by the body in fat cells around the lower part of the body and called on only when the short-term fuel has run out. Might it be that dietary fat (fat that we eat as opposed to make in our own bodies) is more readily laid down to reserve fuel supplies than is sugar?

Whatever the reason, the experience of many women is that a low-fat plan is extremely effective in countering fat bottoms and thighs.

But if this eating plan is to work for you, please be sure that you have diagnosed your overfat problem correctly. Please be honest with yourself about whether your overfat is situated only below the waist and not all over. Also ask yourself whether your too large bottom-half might in fact be due to a swollen belly, and therefore be better attacked through the Anti-candida Eating Plan (p. 228). If you really have got the right diagnosis then this is the beginning of the end of all your problems. The diet is easy to follow, and before long you could be saying goodbye to your cellulite for the first time ever.

HOW IT WORKS

It is very likely that you are starting this eating plan after a history of failures with conventional slimming diets. A quick look round the changing-room at my local gym shows me how many otherwise perfectly slim and fit women have dimply bottoms and flabby thighs. It has to be the despair of every dieter. I believe that the reason conventional slimming diets fail in this area is because they are not specific enough.

An ordinary diet will tell you to cut out a whole range of foods which may not actually be causing you any problems. This broad spectrum approach is also incredibly difficult to stick to on a diet, and when, as you inevitably will, you break the diet, it may well be to eat exactly the foods which are causing you the most problems.

The aim of the Low-fat Eating Plan is to identify exactly which foods are problematic for you and substitute them with other foods. It is easier to stick to because it leaves you with many, many foods that you can eat without worrying. It also shows you which foods to avoid if you are going to break your diet.

You will notice that, contrary to current nutritional thinking, sugary foods are not excluded on the Low-fat Eating Plan. Certainly in an ideal world one would cut back on sugar as well, but as usual in this book we are concerned with reality and the art of the possible. Your symptoms suggest that sugar is not the culprit in your particular overfat problem. Eating too many fatty foods is your problem, rather than too much sugar. So if you can cut fat out of your eating you will have done enough without worrying about sugar as well.

This is the great beauty of the eating plan concept. It is tailor-made for each individual, rather than being a broad generalisation which may not be applicable in a specific case. If you are following a diet which is not truly applicable to your particular case, then you will almost certainly fail on it. By being diagnosed correct for you, the Low-fat Eating Plan carries a much higher chance of success. So good luck and go for it.

STEP-BY-STEP GUIDE TO THE LOW-FAT EATING PLAN

1   Read all sections of the diet carefully.

2   Learn what the stop foods are and why you must stop them.

3   Get familiar with all the substitutes and where to buy them.

4   Go through the week-long sample eating programme and work out how it will fit into your lifestyle.

5   If you are at all uncertain, you can decide to follow the sample eating programme exactly for a week until you get the hang of things.

6   Learn how to make the snack substitutes.

7   Make a copy of the glance guide to stop and substitute foods.

8   Take the glance guide shopping with you to make sure you are stocking up on the right foods.

9   Remember that any food not mentioned as a stop food can be eaten whenever you like.

10   Note which drinks are to be stopped.

11   Eat plenty of fresh vegetables – these are not stop foods.

12   Follow the diet for at least 2 months before reviewing your
      symptoms and deciding whether to continue on it, change to another
      diet, or return to normal eating.

STOP, THINK, SUBSTITUTE

Which foods should I stop eating and what should I substitute?

Complex Carbohydrate Group

Complex carbohydrate is the name nutritionists give to the range
of starchy foods which form the basic staple of the ethnic diet in
nearly every country. They include foods like bread, cereal and
potatoes (until recently the staple over Northern Europe); pasta
(the Mediterranean staple); and rice (the Asian staple).

This food group is aptly called 'complex' because it provides a
complex of nutrients – not just carbohydrate itself but also fibre,
water, vitamins, trace elements and even some protein.

Modern nutritional thinking is that we should partially revert
to peasant eating habits by making complex carbohydrates the
lion's share of the food we eat and therefore the main source of
our calorie intake. Doing this alone would substantially reduce
the amount of fat in the diet because complex carbohydrates
do not naturally contain fat in the way that some protein sources
do. By definition you can't obtain the undesirable animal fat
from a plant product, which is what all complex carbohydrates
are.

So on your low-fat eating plan you should seek to increase
rather than decrease your consumption of complex carbohydrates. But do watch how you prepare them. Don't fry your
bread. Avoid fatty sauces on your pasta. If you are frying rice, use
just a trace of olive oil rather than a large knob of dripping.

● **Stop**: Any cooking of carbohydrates which adds fat, e.g.
  fried bread.

- **Substitute:** Other methods, e.g. toasted bread.

Refined Carbohydrate Group

Refined carbohydrate is complex carbohydrate which has been processed in one of various ways to extract only the main calorie source – sugar – and discard the other components – water, fibre and so on. The refining process turns what is a nutritionally cost-effective dietary source into one that is nutritionally poor value for calories. Certainly, refined carbohydrate yields plenty of energy, but it does not provide any of the other dietary factors the body needs. Whereas you could in fact live (if not well) by bread alone, you could not live by sugar alone.

For the low-fat eating planner this in itself is not a major problem, since your symptoms suggest that what you are eating too much of is not sugar but fat. What causes the problem is the way in which the majority of refined carbohydrate is presented in the modern Western diet – that is, in combination with fat.

Whoever first thought of mixing fat and sugar together has been responsible for so much temptation Satan would be proud. The mixture of animal fat and sugar (with perhaps a little flour and then cooked in some way) proves quite addictive to the vast majority of humans. Nutritionally it is a disaster. Fat and sugar are perhaps the two worst value-for-calorie ingredients in our dietary range. They also have an extremely high calorie density. Add a little cocoa and you've got the dark diet de-railer: chocolate.

So although, as a low-fat eating planner, sugar is not your problem, you are still going to have to forgo all those sugary, fatty, delicious treats.

But don't try to fight your sweet tooth. It's your fat we are fighting, so allow yourself sweet treats like jam or polo mints, as long as they've got no fat with them (if in doubt check the label). You fancy a jam doughnut? Try a hot granary roll with jam and low-fat cottage cheese.

- **Stop**: Biscuits, cakes and pâtisserie which include fat or
  dairy in the recipe, e.g. shortbread, cream buns, etc.;
  croissants; doughnuts; pastry.

- **Substitute**: Granary rolls and variety breads topped with
  honey and cottage cheese or diet fromage frais; meringues
  with low-fat yoghurt; oatcakes; crispbreads; fruit.

Protein Group

Protein is available to us in a wide range of dietary sources
including beans, pulses, rice, eggs, meat, fish and soya bean curd.
Unfortunately, by far the most popular of these sources in the
West is meat. Meat not only naturally contains saturated animal
fat, it is also often cooked in saturated fats.

There are various problems with saturated fat. Like all fats it
is calorie-dense (it contains a comparatively high amount of
calories for its volume). Some nutritionists also believe that it is
difficult to metabolise, especially for women. The British Heart
Foundation is convinced that it contributes to the raising of
blood cholesterol levels, which in turn increases the risk of
arterial and cardiac disease, and recent research has also
indicated that women whose diet is high in animal fat may also
have an increased risk of developing breast cancer.

So animal fat is bad news on three counts: it makes you fat; it
makes you unhealthy; it puts you at risk of disease. For these
reasons the low-fat eating planner must make a major effort to
get protein from sources other than meat as far as possible. There
are plenty of other sources – look at the Vegetarian Eating Plan
(p. 294) to get some ideas.

Lean meat cooked without fat *is* permitted, but I wouldn't
regard it as a daily necessity at all.

- **Stop**: Fried/roast meats; fatty meats; fried fish; sausages;
  pâté; bacon; black pudding; commercial meat products

with a high fat content (e.g. pork pies, Scotch eggs; sausage rolls and many convenience foods and ready meals).

- **Substitute**: Grilled and casseroled lean meats; poached and grilled fish; grilled fish fingers; home-made pies and meals; pulse and bean-based meals; vegetarian products.

Vegetable and Fruit Group

About the only vegetable or fruit that naturally contains a high amount of fat is the avocado. Apart from that, a high content of fresh vegetables and fruit is ideal in the diet of the low-fat eating planner.

Provided they are not overtreated, overstored, or overcooked, fruit and veg are wonderful value for calories. They contain fibre, water, vitamins and trace elements as well as carbohydrate. They also have a very high degree of flavour, which if they are sensitively cooked, goes a long way towards preventing a planned eater becoming bored or suffering from cravings.

Some recent research has also suggested that the soluble fibre present in many fruits and vegetables may also prevent fatty deposits being laid down in the bloodstream. The idea is that the fibre traps the fat molecules during digestion and carries them with it when it is excreted from the system. As you know, fibre is largely excreted rather than wholly digested. Soluble fibre (you can identify it because it dissolves in water and forms a sort of sticky goo) is believed to do this more effectively than non-soluble fibre (like bran) because it goes through the system more quickly. This thinking may yet be disproved, but in case it is eventually corroborated it's a good idea to include plenty of soluble fibre in your diet.

- **Stop**: Deep-fried vegetables (chips, onion-rings, etc.); potato crisps; avocado pears.

- **Substitute**: Stir-fried and grilled vegetables; steamed and raw vegetables; olives/raisins.

Dairy Group

Dairy products are made from animal fats, and while many nutritionists now favour dairy products, the low-fat eating planner cannot afford this source of fat in the diet – particularly when there are plenty of low-fat dairy alternatives.

- **Stop**: Full cream milk; butter; cream; cheese; chocolates; whole milk shakes and malted drinks.

- **Substitute**: Skimmed milk; low-fat spread; yoghurt/fromage frais; cottage cheese; yoghurt shakes.

Fats Group

As we have discussed, saturated animal fats are on the Stop list. But what about polyunsaturated fats, which we hear so much about? Polyunsaturated fats and oils may well be healthier than saturated fats, but they are not lower in calories. Many people are fooled into thinking that a polyunsaturated vegetable margarine is less fatty and has fewer calories than the same amount of butter. It does not.

Moreover, some criticisms have recently been levelled at the methods of processing and ingredients used in making polyunsaturated vegetable margarines and oils. Whether or not these are accurate, there is no doubt that the vegetable polyunsaturated fats are more highly processed than butter.

When choosing my own oil/fat my personal preference is for first cold-pressed virgin olive oil. This is a mono-unsaturated oil which many nutritionists believe to be the most healthy of all. Some even believe that its role in the Mediterranean diet may be a preventative against heart disease. A realist would say that the reason fewer people die from heart disease in the Mediterranean countries is because they have died from cancer first, but it's as well to take all the current thinking into account. The main reason I use extra virgin oil is because it tastes so delicious! I need use only a tiny quantity of it and I never end up craving for some other fat. In Italian restaurants you are given a little dish of it to dip your ciabatta bread into and it is scrumptious.

- **Stop:** Lard; dripping; butter; saturated oils.
- **Substitute:** Sparing olive oil for stir-frying; low-fat spread for butter; tomato juice/lemon juice/vinegar for sauces, sautéing, moistening, etc.

Condiments

Obviously the fattier your gravy the more care you need to take to strain it or prepare it in a different method. Never, never add fat to your gravy pan. Don't use a roux to thicken. You can either reduce the sauce like the French do by boiling vigorously, or you can mix a little cold stock and cornflour and then stir that into the pan.

- **Stop:** Gravy.
- **Substitute:** Pan juice reductions, vegetables or tomato purée.

Beverages

The simple guide with drinks is – if it's got full cream milk in it, switch to something else. You don't need to worry about sugary drinks.

- **Stop:** Milky drinks.
- **Substitute:** Skimmed milk/yoghurt-based drinks.

Eating Out and Take-away

When eating out these days there are nearly always good low-fat options on the menu. Some restaurants even put a special asterisk against their low-fat options so that you can spot them easily. So many businessmen have been told to reduce fat in order to lower their cholesterol that restaurants would be very foolish indeed not to provide them with something to eat. Ask the waiter to recommend a low-fat dish.

If the restaurant is unenlightened you can still do fine. Choose a fruit or salad-based starter or a soup. For the main course choose a grilled lean meat or fish with plenty of vegetables, salad, and baked, boiled or mashed potatoes. Dessert can be fruit, jelly, meringue (but not cream).

Some forms of take-away are fattier than others, so you can compromise. Fried fish and chips are off limits, but the same chippy may do a meat pie and baked potato which, while not fat-free, is much lower in fat.

Indian take-away can be pretty fatty – even the breads are often fried. Choose chapatti rather than nan or poppadom. Choose tandoor-roast dishes rather than pasandas and biryanis. Basically, if it looks greasy, it's fatty.

Greek take-away is usually chargrilled and free from fatty sauces. The oil used in cooking should also be olive oil. If it's not olive oil they're not real Greeks. Choose a grilled lamb or chicken kebab in pitta bread with salad. Dolmades (stuffed vine leaves) are great, but avoid taramasalata (have tzatsiki instead) and the heavy dishes like moussaka and stifado.

Chinese take-away is a minefield, as every Chinese chef cooks differently. Minimise the damage by opting for stir-fried rather than deep-fried dishes; seafood and vegetables rather than duck and meat; boiled rice rather than fried rice.

If you've ever eaten a real Italian pizza you'll realise what a travesty the ones you get in Britain are. Instead of being a crisp nutritious mix of complex carbohydrates and vegetables with a little garnish of cheese or meat, they are mammoth, fatty, gooey dumplings with the healthy tomato purée more or less non-existent and the fatty cheese topping swollen out of proportion.

Enough said. Enough said too about burgers and shakes. Burgers are OK if they really are made of excellent beef well-grilled over a flame and served in a granary bun without cheese or butter. The shakes you can stand your toddler upright in are never OK, ever, for anyone.

AT-A-GLANCE GUIDE TO
STOP AND SUBSTITUTE FOODS

Stop – *Substitute*

Complex Carbohydrate Food Group

fried bread – *toast*

Refined Carbohydrate Food Group

croissants – *hot granary rolls*

biscuits – *oatcakes/crispbread*

doughnuts – *bread roll with honey/jam and cottage cheese*

pâtisserie – *meringues (no cream)*

cakes – *fruit and fromage frais*

pancakes – *grilled potato cakes with syrup*

pastry – *mashed potato/crumbled Ryvita/oatcake as appropriate*

Protein Food Group

fried/roast meats – *grilled/sautéd meats*

deep fried fish – *poached/grilled fish*

sausages – *grilled fish fingers*

pâté – *Marmite/Bovril*

commercial pies and meals – *fish pie/ home-made stew*

black pudding – *haggis/potato farls*

bacon – *grilled continental ham*

peanuts – *olives/raisins/cocktail pickles*

taramasalata – *tzatsiki (cucumber blended with yoghurt)*

Scotch egg – *hard-boiled egg (or remove coating)*

pork pie – *ham sandwich*

fatty meats – *lean meats*

Indian take-away – *Greek take-away*

Vegetable and Fruit Food Group

chips – *stir-fried carrot and parsnip sticks*

roast potatoes – *baked/boiled/mashed potatoes*

potato crisps – *olives/raisins/cocktail pickles*

avocado pears – *aubergines*

fried onions – *grilled tomatoes*

Dairy Food Group

milk – *skimmed milk*

cream – *yoghurt*

cheese – *cottage cheese*

chocolates – *banana/Ryvita sandwich*

Fats Group

butter – *low fat spread*

fats – *olive oil (sparing)*

frying oils – *tomato juice/lemon juice/vinegar*

Condiments

gravy – *tomato sauce/pan juice reduction*

SAMPLE SUBSTITUTION PROGRAMME

* Items marked with an asterisk are given in greater detail in the Snack Substitutes and Recipes sections (pp. 313, 324).

MONDAY

Breakfast

Normal Croissant with butter and marmalade; cereal with milk; fresh unsweetened orange juice; coffee with milk

Includes these Stop Foods Croissant, butter, whole milk

Substitute 2 slices soda bread toast with low-fat spread and marmalade; cereal with skimmed milk; fresh squeezed unsweetened orange juice; black coffee

Elevenses

Normal I biscuit; coffee with milk, no sugar

Stop Biscuit, whole milk

Substitute *I plain oatcake; black coffee

Lunch

Normal Pâté on buttered toast; sausage and chips; apple; I glass wine

Stop Pâté, butter, sausage, chips

Substitute Large bowl of soup with 2 slices of toast, Bovril, no butter; large ham salad and baked potato with cottage cheese, no butter; apple; I glass wine

Afternoon tea

Normal Piece of cake; cup of tea without sugar

Stop Cake

Substitute *2 rice cakes spread with flavoured diet fromage frais; cup of tea

Dinner

Normal Prawn cocktail with 2 slices brown bread and butter; pasta in cheese sauce with courgettes; ice-cream

Stop Butter, cheese, ice-cream

Substitute Prawn cocktail with 2 slices brown bread and low-fat spread; *pasta in tomato sauce with courgettes; *plain low-fat yoghurt mashed with frozen raspberries

TUESDAY

Breakfast

Normal 2 fried eggs on buttered toast; fresh orange juice; coffee

Stop Fried egg, butter

Substitute 2 poached eggs on toast with low-fat spread; fresh orange juice; coffee

Elevenses

Normal American-style cookie; coffee

Stop Cookie

Substitute Orange; coffee

Lunch

Normal Fried chicken limb in breadcrumbs; chips; peas; individual portion fruit trifle; glass wine; coffee

Stop Fried chicken, chips, trifle

Substitute Grilled chicken with large salad (*vinaigrette dressing) and bread roll (no butter); fruit salad with yoghurt; sparkling mineral water; coffee

Afternoon tea

Normal Small bar of chocolate; tea

Stop Chocolate

Substitute *Banana and Ryvita sandwich

Dinner

Normal Packet of potato crisps; sausages; baked beans; 2 slices buttered toast; flavoured jelly; 2 glasses wine; coffee; 1 chocolate truffle

Stop Potato crisps, sausages, butter, truffle

Substitute *Handful of black olives and cocktail pickles; grilled fish fingers; 2 slices toast with low-fat spread; baked beans; flavoured jelly; 2 glasses wine; coffee; tangerine

WEDNESDAY

Breakfast

Normal Cereal with milk; pancake with maple syrup; fresh squeezed orange juice; coffee

Stop Whole milk; fat for frying

Substitute Cereal with skimmed milk; pancake mixture made with skimmed milk and fried in a non-stick pan with smear of olive oil; fresh squeezed orange juice; coffee

Elevenses

Normal Shortcake biscuit; coffee

Stop Shortcake biscuit

Substitute *Rice cake spread with flavoured cottage cheese; coffee

Lunch

Normal Scotch egg salad; 2 slices brown bread and butter; apple; wine; coffee

Stop Scotch egg, butter

Substitute Ham sandwich (no butter); large continental salad; apple; wine; coffee

Afternoon tea

Normal Snack bar; tea

Stop Snack bar

Substitute *Oatcake; tea

Dinner

Normal Bowl of soup; grilled lamb chop; spinach; mashed potato; tinned tomato; fresh unsugared fruit salad; coffee

Stop None

Substitute None

THURSDAY

Breakfast

Normal 2 rashers of bacon and 1 fried egg on toast; fresh orange juice; black coffee

Stop Bacon, fried egg

Substitute Continental breakfast of 1 hard-boiled egg; 1 slice ham; 1 bread roll with cottage cheese (no butter); fresh orange juice; coffee

Elevenses

Normal Chocolate digestive biscuit; coffee

Stop Biscuit

Substitute *2 Ryvitas spread with honey and flavoured cottage cheese; coffee

Lunch

Normal Fried fish and chips; peas; chocolate gâteau; coffee; Coca Cola
Stop Fried fish, chips, chocolate gâteau
Substitute Grilled/poached fish; boiled potatoes (no butter); peas; salad;
*mashed banana with yoghurt and crumbled oatcake; coffee; Coca Cola

Afternoon tea

Normal Egg sandwich; tea
Stop Butter, mayonnaise
Substitute Salad sandwich on brown bread, no butter, no mayonnaise; tea

Dinner

Normal Taramasalata with brown bread and butter; commercially prepared
minced beef pie; gravy; sautéd potatoes; fried onions; ice-cream; 2 glasses wine;
coffee; after-dinner mint
Stop Taramasalata, butter, commercially prepared meal, gravy, sautéd potatoes, fried onions, ice-cream
Substitute *Tzatsiki with pitta bread (no butter); *home-made beef casserole
with no added fat (or commercially prepared meal if ingredients contain no
more than 20 per cent fat); *thin tomato purée heated; mashed potato; onions
quartered and grilled; *frozen yoghurt; 2 glasses wine; mint

FRIDAY

Breakfast

Normal Toast with butter and jam; coffee with skimmed milk
Stop Butter
Substitute Toast with low-fat spread and jam; coffee with skimmed milk

Elevenses

Normal Apple; black coffee
Stop None
Substitute None

Lunch

Normal Pork pie with chutney; tomato salad; 2 glasses wine; coffee
Stop Pork pie
Substitute *Tuna salad; tomato salad; 2 glasses wine; coffee

Afternoon tea

Normal Ginger biscuit; tea
Stop Ginger biscuit
Substitute *Ryvita and flavoured cottage cheese; tea

Dinner

Normal 3 measures spirit; Indian take-away; 2 glasses wine; coffee; mint
Stop Indian take-away
Substitute 3 measures spirit (if you must); Greek take-away (not taramasalata); 2 glasses wine; coffee; mint

SATURDAY

Breakfast

Normal 1 slice buttered toast; coffee with skimmed milk
Stop Butter
Substitute Toast with low-fat spread and Marmite; coffee; sparkling mineral water

Elevenses

Normal Doughnut; coffee
Stop Doughnut
Substitute Egg custard tart; coffee. While not completely fat-free, at least the egg custard has not been fried and therefore presents a good weekend compromise!

Lunch

Normal Pub lunch of bread, butter, cheese, chutney, salad, chips; ½ pint shandy

Stop Butter, cheese, chips
Substitute Pub lunch of gammon with pineapple; salad; shandy

Afternoon tea

Normal Cake; tea
Stop Cake
Substitute *Honey and cottage cheese sandwiches made with soda bread; tea

Dinner

Normal 2 measures spirit; avocado filled with prawns; well-grilled steak; peas; baked potato with butter; grilled tomatoes and mushrooms; ice-cream; 3 glasses wine
Stop Avocado, butter, ice-cream
Substitute 2 measures spirit (it is Saturday, after all); *plain seafood salad; steak; peas; baked potato with low-fat spread or cottage cheese; grilled tomatoes and mushrooms; fresh fruit salad; sparkling mineral water

SUNDAY

Breakfast

Normal Bacon; sausage; fried bread; grilled tomatoes; orange juice; black coffee
Stop Bacon, sausage, fried bread
Substitute Herb-flavoured scrambled egg on toast with grilled tomatoes and grilled mushrooms; fresh squeezed orange juice; coffee

No elevenses today

Lunch

Normal 2 measures spirit; roast pork; roast potatoes; cabbage; peas; gravy; apple pie with cream; coffee with skimmed milk
Stop Roast pork, roast potatoes, gravy, cream
Substitute 2 measures spirit; grilled pork chops (fat removed) with tomato and mustard sauce; mashed potato; cabbage; peas; apple pie with yoghurt or low-fat fromage frais; coffee

Afternoon tea

Normal Biscuit; tea
Stop Biscuit
Substitute 1 slice toasted soda bread with honey; tea

Dinner

Normal Spanish omelette; salad; bread; cheese; celery; 2 glasses wine
Stop Cheese
Substitute Spanish omelette; salad; bread with Marmite and cottage cheese; celery; 2 glasses wine

WHAT NEXT?

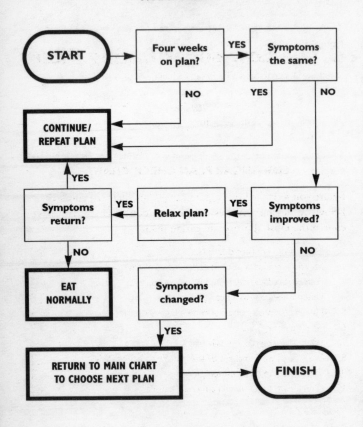

3. The Low-sugar Eating Plan

LOW-SUGAR PLAN CHECK CHART

Before you start the Low-sugar Eating Plan, fill in the check chart below by ticking any Yes answers to double-check you have chosen the most appropriate eating plan.

1. I suffer from bouts of dizziness. ☐
2. My concentration is poor at certain times of day. ☐
3. I can get tired and depressed for no reason. ☐
4. I often wake up with a headache. ☐
5. My symptoms only occur at certain times of the month. ☐
6. I don't eat very much. ☐
7. When I break a diet I usually binge. ☐
8. The hours I work make it difficult for me to eat healthily. ☐
9. Chocolate is my greatest temptation. ☐
10. I find it hard to tell when I am really hungry. ☐

Ticks KEY

0–3 It is unlikely that the Low-sugar Eating Plan is the right answer for you. Return to the Eating Plan Map (pp. 12–13) and follow the arrows further.

4–8 Your symptoms suggest fluctuating blood-sugar levels and a borderline eating disorder which will respond to the Low-sugar Eating Plan. If you know you have an eating disorder read the Eating Disorder section before you start the Low-sugar Eating Plan.

9–10 Your results point to a generally poor level of nutrition. Check out the Low-processing Eating Plan to see if it is more appropriate.

IMPORTANT: If you answered Yes to 5, go to the sections dealing with the menstrual and oral contraceptive syndromes (pp. 181, 207).

WELCOME TO THE LOW-SUGAR EATING PLAN

Since you've chosen the Low-sugar Eating Plan, I'm willing to bet that you are reckoning to start the plan, which you think of as 'The Diet', on Monday morning. And you're probably looking forward to having a good binge at the weekend, treating yourself to all the nice things you won't be able to eat while you're on the eating plan. And how many times before have you said all this to yourself?

I've got news for you. It's too late to have your normal pre-diet pig-out, because you are already on the Low-sugar Eating Plan. From the moment you correctly diagnosed your eating problem and began reading this section, you took the first step on the road that is going to solve your over-fat and dieting difficulties permanently.

So the bad news is that you will already be on the Low-sugar Eating Plan this weekend. But here's the good news. It doesn't mean you won't be able to have a binge. You can eat as much as you like this weekend — and some of it can be what you might think of as 'bad' foods like fish and chips; peanuts; bacon butties and the like.

The Low-sugar Eating Plan is a very special nutritional programme designed specifically to deal with a problem that undermines very many efforts at fat loss. I've christened it the Monday Syndrome. I've already hinted at pretty much what the Monday Syndrome is, and as you almost certainly suffer from it you could probably write a good description of it yourself. The

Monday Syndrome really begins the weekend before, when you indulge in all your favourite 'sinful' foods.

Then on Monday morning you wake up with the most wonderful optimistic feeling. Today is going to be the first day of the rest of your life. Today is the day you begin The Diet – that special one that's going to be different from all the rest. This is the one that is going to succeed. From today onwards you will begin on the course that will make you thin, tall, beautiful, popular and successful.

As you skip breakfast and lunch the sensation is almost euphoric. There is a very real hope that your whole life is about to change. Or is it? At around 4 in the afternoon the doubts begin to set in. You have now gone for about 20 hours without eating and you haven't turned into Kate Moss. Also, although 20 hours is a long time to go without eating you begin to realise it is nothing like as long as the rest of your life.

On top of these doubts, you suddenly begin to realise that the sensation of optimism and euphoria has subsided. You actually feel inexplicably depressed, and now you come to think of it, very tired and headachey. In fact you really are feeling so low that you simply must have something to eat. But it is too late for lunch and too early for dinner, so you can't have a meal, and anyway, you are on The Diet. So you opt just to have a snack. A cup of coffee and a bar of chocolate will keep you going until dinner time and a little snack like that can't harm your diet because you've already missed breakfast and lunch.

After the snack you feel better, and excited again at how well the diet is going. It's perhaps an hour later when you get up quickly and your head swims. You feel so dizzy you might faint. Well, it's nearly evening now, so perhaps just a couple of biscuits or a doughnut from the snack bar to eat on the train home. The tasty snack really gets your appetite going, by the time you are home, you are starving. So you pick at things while you are making the dinner. You congratulate yourself on your wonderful low-calorie meal, but by the end of the evening you are still feeling unsatisfied so you have a piece of left-over apple pie and a cup of coffee with News at Ten.

In bed you review day one of The Diet and are horrified to realise that you ate almost as much as on Sunday. Yes, you skipped breakfast and lunch, but there was the bar (well two bars really) of chocolate, the doughnut, the extra piece of apple pie and a few chocolate mints you had in front of the telly, now you come to think of it. And you did allow yourself quite a large dinner because it was your only proper meal of the day.

Oh, well, there's always next Monday. Then it really will work. On Monday I really will start to be slim and better in every way. And here we go again.

But before you cringe too much in horror at recognising yourself in this scenario, a lot of it isn't your fault. It is not your lack of self-discipline that is to blame, but a biological cycle that your body is being put through by The Diet. Yes, it's really The Diet's fault all along.

Monday Syndrome sufferers tend to develop a form of reactive hypoglycaemia connected with the process by which our bodies metabolise sugars. When we fast for too long after a prolonged feast the level of sugar in our blood falls. When it falls too low the adrenal glands release adrenalin in an effort to raise blood sugar levels. This carries side effects of dizziness; depression; bad temper and moodiness; migraine. If we then pick a sugary food to try to soothe these unpleasant symptoms, the body quickly receives an extra shot of sugar. Together with the adrenalin-triggered raising of blood sugar levels this means that the body is rapidly overloaded.

The now too-high blood sugar level means that insulin is released by the pancreas in order to lower the levels. But because of the double surge, it is likely that the pancreas will be over-stimulated and release too much insulin, causing the blood sugar level to plummet rapidly, and end up too low again. So the vicious circle begins once more.

Nutritionists now believe that this reactive hypoglycaemic vicious circle is at the heart of many eating problems. Monday Syndrome is the most obvious, but bulimics too are likely to be hypoglycaemic.

The pattern is also mirrored in our emotional attitude towards eating and dieting. Nearly all of us who become overfat have done so by eating incorrectly or by overeating. One of the major causes of overeating is emotional deprivation. We feel unhappy for some reason, possibly subconscious, so we eat to cheer ourselves up. By then commencing a conventional slim- ming diet we deprive ourselves of the food we have been using to alleviate our original emotional deprivation. But the emotional deprivation still exists, so we end up doubly deprived: of both emotion and comforting food. This creates the biological and emotional vicious circle that leads to the yo-yo dieting which is so frowned upon.

I used to have Monday Syndrome and rapidly became prone to hypoglycaemia. This went on for quite a few years until the crunch came that forced me out of my bad habit. I became woman's editor of my newspaper, and a 10-hour day turned into 12–14 hours non-stop. As usual I ate neither breakfast nor lunch, but the difference this time was that I no longer had the opportunity to compensate by eating snacks and big dinners. There just wasn't time. When I arrived home in the evenings I just fell into bed without eating. I would wake up in the morning with a savage headache and rush to work without breakfast, because of course I never had breakfast. At the weekends I ate a little, but I was usually too tired and headachey to have much appetite.

My fat and my clothes were falling off me. Even I realised I didn't need to diet any longer. So I came off my diet. I still didn't have time to eat much, but gradually I began to feel better and my weight stabilised. Then I realised that I was actually eating quite differently from how I had before. When I did eat I didn't worry about what it was that I ate because I was no longer on The Diet, and I gradually realised that the things I preferred to eat were not sugary at all. When I was on The Diet, if I had something to eat it was always a snack like a biscuit or a piece of chocolate because that only felt like 'a little something' and gave a quick energy boost. I wouldn't have dared have a portion of chips or a packet of crisps because they were real 'baddies'.

Once I no longer needed to diet and could have the 'baddies', I preferred to eat them to biscuits. But the difference was that if I had a savoury 'baddy' I generally felt more satisfied and comfortable and would forget completely about eating or picking again until a natural meal break came up.

Although my foods had changed quite a bit, I remained slim. I put this down to the pressures of work. When I left my job in order to write this book I was much less pressurised and within easy reach of the kitchen. Would the fat creep back?

Nearly a year later it has not done so. Now that I am no longer on The Diet I suddenly find I think about food hardly at all. I have my breakfast: 'baddies' like toast with butter or bacon. Then at lunchtime I have lunch. Then at dinner time I have dinner. And that's all there is to it!

I know it sounds quite impossible, but nutritionists back me up. It turns out that quite by chance I had learnt how to break out of my own hypoglycaemic vicious circle. I had done it, not by a conventional slimming diet, but by simply altering my eating habits, by substituting one set of foods for another set. My own personal experience had shown that the policy of food substitution, as opposed to food deprivation, is the way forward for diets.

Simply by substituting foods low in sugar instead of those high in sugar (regardless of their calorie value) you can break the Monday Syndrome and succeed in losing fat. Read on to find out how the Low-sugar Eating Plan works.

HOW IT WORKS

The Low-sugar Eating Plan breaks with conventional slimming diets, and indeed current nutrition advice, in various ways. Like all the eating plans in this book the main point is that this one is tailored to solve a very specific set of problems. It addresses only these problems, rather than setting out to be a cure-all for symptoms that might well not exist in the particular individual who has chosen the plan.

For example, the Low-sugar Eating Plan is not particularly low in calories. Nor, against current guidelines, is it low in fat or salt. The point is that the individual dieter who has chosen the Low-sugar Eating Plan has a problem with sugar specifically, not necessarily with calories or fat or salt. Only by concentrating all our fire on that one particular area can we get a good chance of solving it.

It is unhelpful to take a scattergun approach, with dietary remedies for a whole host of issues from which the eating-planner may or may not suffer. This simply distracts attention from the real problem. And it may eventually undermine the plan.

For example, when the moment comes to snack, if chocolate and potato crisps are equally forbidden, the person with a sugar problem who decides to break the rules will break them with chocolate, not potato crisps. This is the worst thing they could do, because it will set off the reactive hypoglycaemic vicious circle. Potato crisps would have been much less harmful, because although a little fatty and salty, they contain virtually no sugar (and incidentally, fewer calories).

Therefore the Low-sugar Eating Plan does not forbid foods such as potato crisps, and when the time comes for a snack, for something 'a bit bad', crisps can offer themselves as a suitable compromise. On a conventional slimming diet the person with a sugar problem would find them both banned and opt for chocolate.

Throughout these eating plans you will repeatedly find the compromise option taken. The practical expedient that will actually work is what we are looking for, rather than the ideal solution which is in the end not achieved. So the Low-sugar Eating Plan concentrates specifically on reducing the amount of sugar in your diet and lets the rest take care of itself.

When you have cured your sugar problem you are very likely to find that you have no other problems. But you may discover hidden ones that, although not as important as the sugar problem, are now more apparent.

For example, if you were overfat everywhere before and lose fat on the Low-sugar Eating Plan you may find that your thighs remain overfat, which would suggest you try a period on the Low-fat Eating Plan (p. 74). Or it might be that your blood cholesterol level remains high (though this is unlikely) so that you would want to move on to the Low-cholesterol Eating Plan (p. 129).

That is why I suggest that you return to the Eating Plans Map (pp. 12–13) once you have successfully completed a plan. But of all the plans in this book, I am confident that the Low-sugar Eating Plan will help you beat a specific problem and that you will have no more difficulties with eating or overfat.

STEP-BY-STEP GUIDE TO THE LOW-SUGAR EATING PLAN

1   Read all sections of the diet carefully.

2   Learn what the stop foods are and why you must stop them.

3   Get familiar with all the substitutes and where to buy them.

4   Go through the week-long sample eating programme and work out how it will fit into your lifestyle.

5   If you are at all uncertain you can decide to follow the sample eating programme exactly for a week until you get the hang of things.

6   Learn how to make the snack substitutes.

7   Make a copy of the glance guide to stop and substitute foods.

8   Take the glance guide shopping with you to make sure you are stocking up on the right foods.

9   Remember that any food not mentioned as a stop food can be eaten whenever you like.

10   Note which drinks are to be stopped.

11   Eat plenty of fresh vegetables, these are not stop foods.

12   Follow the diet for a month before reviewing your symptoms and deciding whether to continue on it, change to another diet, or return to normal eating.

STOP, THINK, SUBSTITUTE

Which foods should I stop eating and what should I substitute with?

Complex Carbohydrate Group

Complex carbohydrate is basically sugar that comes along with a whole complex of other dietary components – fibre, water, vitamins, minerals, trace elements, some protein – all bound together in a single food product. The complex carbohydrate foods are: cereals (oats, maize, wheat, rye, etc.) and the products made from them (bread, pasta, flour); roots (potatoes, beet, etc.); rice (a cereal crop but unusual in being comparatively high in protein).

Even though you are on the Low-sugar Eating Plan, complex carbohydrate is not a problem for you because it is nutritionally different from refined carbohydrate, which is sugar stripped of the rest of its dietary components. You can easily tell the dietary difference between a complex and a refined carbohydrate product: the complex carbohydrate product will not taste particularly sweet, whereas the refined carbohydrate product will have a sweet taste.

As someone with a sugar problem it is very likely that the root of your difficulty is the sweet taste and instant energy buzz obtained from refined carbohydrate. You may have become more or less addicted to this sweet rush, and therefore the more refined carbohydrate you eat, the more you will want to eat. The sweet rush is not obtained from complex carbohydrate, so it will not feed your addiction. But to begin with you should beware of complex carbohydrates that are very quickly broken down or 'refined' by your body's own digestive system.

A simple experiment to discover this process is to put an ordinary piece of white factory bread in your mouth and chew it for a few moments without swallowing. Almost immediately it begins to taste sweet. That is because your saliva contains an enzyme which rapidly releases the sugar in white bread, long before the digestive process begins in the stomach and gut. Opting for brown bread will slow this down a bit.

- **Stop**: White bread.

- **Substitute**: Brown bread.

Refined Carbohydrate Group

As we learnt in the section above, refined carbohydrates are the main problem for the low-sugar eating planner. The basic refined carbohydrate is common white sugar. It is refined from complex carbohydrate sources – usually sugar beet or sugar cane. The refining process strips away the complex of other dietary ingredients (fibre, water, vitamins, minerals, etc.) and leaves the simple sugar, which is purely a unit of calorific energy without other nutritional ingredients.

A simple sugar can be refined from many different plant-origin complex carbohydrates, but the basic result is always the same: sugar. The different sugars have lots of different names – glucose, sucrose, malt, etc. – but they all amount to much the same thing.

Whatever the marketing men may try to tell you, no particular sugar is better for you than any other. Neither, to be brutally honest, is honey, even though I have listed it as an alternative here. Honey is simply a sugar that has been refined from plant matter by bees in a factory called a beehive.

Logically speaking, honey should be just as addictive as any other refined carbohydrate, but it does not seem to have quite that effect on human psychology. Very often sugar addicts find honey is a successful intermediate step in going cold turkey from sugar. For some reason when low-sugar eating planners substitute honey for sugar they don't seem to use as much, nor to become as dependent on it as on sugar. I don't know why this is – ask the bees.

So when you begin your Low-sugar Eating Plan, start by substituting honey sparingly as a spread and sweetener. It may not work with you, in which case you will have to give up honey as well, but for most people it seems to.

- **Stop:** Sugar, syrup, treacle, molasses, sweetened breakfast cereal (check label); sweets, cakes; biscuits; commercial puddings and desserts; doughnuts; pâtisserie.

- **Substitute:** Use honey sparingly instead of any sugar product, or use fruit juice for sweetening in cooking; porridge; eat crisps and nuts instead of sweet snacks; wholemeal bread rolls with cheese/cream cheese instead of cakes; crispbreads, toast for biscuits; fresh fruit/yoghurt for puddings.

Protein Group

While carbohydrates are eventually broken down by the body into sugars to be used for fuel, proteins follow a different digestive path. The digestive enzyme pepsin acts on protein to provide peptone, an intermediate form, which is eventually broken down into amino acids called peptides.

These amino acids form building blocks to manufacture muscle and other body tissues, including blood and enzymes. Amino acids are only burnt as fuel if there aren't any other fuel sources (e.g. carbohydrate) around. So you can think of protein and carbohydrate as two different kinds of wood. Protein is the sort of wood you use for building a log cabin or a table; carbohydrate is the sort of wood you put on the fire. You don't burn the table unless you've run out of firewood. Similarly the body only burns amino acid as energy for two reasons: it does not have enough carbohydrate fuel; or it has plenty of amino acid fuel to spare.

So unless you are a protein addict as well as a sugar addict (in fact people are usually one or the other), protein energy is not the same problem for a low-sugar eating planner as sugar energy is. The only thing you really need to watch about your protein intake is that it is not coming to you laced with refined sugar.

- **Stop**: Sweetened baked beans (check label); convenience foods containing sugar (check label).

- **Substitute**: Health food baked beans (available in supermarkets); home-made meals as far as possible.

Vegetable and Fruit Group

Fruits have an ambivalent position in the diet of a low-sugar eating planner because they contain simple carbohydrates, which fall between the two other types. They have not been processed in the way that refined carbohydrates have, but all the same the sugars that simple carbohydrates contain are more readily available to be metabolised by the body than those in complex carbohydrates.

Again, the taste test helps. Fruits aren't as sweet as sugary foods, but they are sweeter than grain foods. So does this mean that the low-sugar eating planner should steer clear of them? Yes, but not necessarily completely. Experiment by eating various different fruits. Bananas are excellent, in that they are not too sweet and sugary and have some useful vitamin and trace elements. I find that because of their high water content fresh fruits are not generally too much of a threat – but beware of dried fruit.

- **Stop**: High sugar fruits (dried fruit, melons, etc.); sweetened tinned fruit; tinned vegetables containing sugar (check label); sweetened fruit juices and squashes.

- **Substitute**: Lower sugar fruits (bananas, apricots, etc.); fresh fruit or unsweetened tinned fruit; raw vegetables; unsweetened fresh fruit juice.

Dairy Group

As a low-sugar eating planner you will know that probably the most dangerous food of all for you is chocolate. It really is a fairly addictive concoction. Sugar, caffeine and theobromine give you a 'rush'. Dairy fat content gives what the marketing men call 'mouth appeal'. Cocoa gives a unique taste which is not replicated elsewhere in our diet.

All these things make chocolate difficult not only to give up but also to substitute in your eating plan. But chocolate must be stopped, as we have discovered at the beginning of this eating plan.

Psychologically chocolate is a 'treat' food. It is not nutritionally necessary to us, but for many people it is a mood enhancer. Therefore when we seek to substitute chocolate it is important to substitute it with a food that is equally perceived to be a 'treat' food rather than a healthy food.

This is where many diets go wrong. They tell you to eat carrot sticks when you need a bar of chocolate. Everybody's treat foods are different, so I have not been too specific about what you should substitute chocolate with. Obviously it must be one of your other treat foods, but as you are a low-sugar eating planner that food must not contain sugar.

So think of the naughtiest food you can imagine. It can be anything at all: chips; cream cheese; pâté de foie gras. The only rule – and I mean this, forget about calories or fat or salt or whatever – is that it must not contain sugar. For me the ultimate naughty treat is a packet of cheese and onion flavoured potato crisps.

- **Stop**: Chocolate; malted drinks; sweetened milk shakes; ice-creams and sorbets.

- **Substitute**: Banana and cream cheese on oatcake/cheese/ crisps (any flavour); milk with vanilla extract; fruit juice and yoghurt shake; frozen yoghurt/chilled fruit.

Fats Group

The thinking behind planned eating is that you address one dietary problem at a time until you know exactly where you are. Through the diagnosis methods in this book you have discovered that too high an intake of sugar is your primary problem. So concentrate on addressing this rather than anything else.

You will read a lot about how bad for you fat is. Perhaps this should be how bad it is for one in general. We are all individuals. Fat may be your next door neighbour's biggest enemy, but that doesn't mean it's yours.

Let's get this sugar problem licked and then we'll think about fat. Don't persecute yourself trying to give up fat as well as sugar.

Condiments

The simple rule with condiments is to look at the label and if it contains sugar, or anything that sounds like sugar (see the section on how to read a label, p. 14), replace it with something that doesn't contain sugar.

- **Stop**: Jam, syrup; tomato ketchup; dessert toppings; pre-prepared sauces.

- **Substitute**: Marmite/Bovril; home-made tomato purée; whipped cream; home-made sauces.

Beverages

Anybody who has ever shopped in a supermarket will know that there are now 'diet' versions available of most popular colas and soft drinks. These usually use Nutrasweet as a non-sugar sweetener.

I am a great fan of Nutrasweet. I think it tastes just as good as sugar and since nobody so far has managed to prove that it might be a carcinogen, I can't see a good reason for ever having sugar again.

But for a low-sugar eating planner, as opposed to those on any other eating plan, one of the aims is to cure you of your sweet tooth. Simply substituting Nutrasweet for sugar is not going to do that, so for the time being at least, you must cut out diet colas and soft drinks as well as ordinary ones.

- **Stop**: Colas, fizzy drinks; sweetened cordial and squashes.

- **Substitute**: Mineral water; tomato juice; fresh fruit juice.

Eating Out and Take-away

Eating out and take-aways are not so much of a problem for those on the Low-sugar Eating Plan as for those on other plans like low-fat (p. 74) and low-cholesterol (p. 129). For one thing, it is generally quite easy to spot if something contains sugar because it tastes sweet. So whether you are eating out or taking-away, avoid sweet foods (including dishes like Chinese sweet and sour). As with convenience foods, many savoury dishes do in fact contain sugar, so try to avoid these as far as possible by choosing plainer dishes rather than those with rich sauces or complicated sounding names and recipes. When it comes to dessert you have the luxury of being able to have the cheese board instead of the chocolate gâteau. Just think of those poor low-calorie or low-fat eating planners who can't have either!

AT-A-GLANCE GUIDE TO STOP AND SUBSTITUTE FOODS

Stop – *Substitute*

Complex Carbohydrate Food Group

white bread – *granary bread*

Refined Carbohydrate Food Group

biscuits – *potato crisps*
sugar – *honey*
syrup – *unsweetened fruit juice/honey*
cakes – *sandwiches*
commercial puddings and desserts – *yoghurt and fruit*

doughnuts – *wholemeal roll with cheese*
pâtisserie – *toast with cream cheese*
sweetened breakfast cereal – *porridge*
all confectionery – *nuts*

Protein Food Group

sweet and sour dishes – *stir fried meat and vegetables*
baked beans – *unsweetened baked beans (or home-made)*
certain convenience foods (if containing sugar check label) – *plain savoury dishes*

Vegetable and Fruit Food Group

pineapples – *bananas*

dried fruits – *nuts/raw vegetables*

melons – *plums/peaches*

beetroot – *carrots*

strawberries – *cherries*

fruit juices and drinks – *mineral water*

tinned fruit – *fresh bananas*

tinned vegetables – *fresh raw vegetables*

Dairy Food Group

chocolate – *banana and cream cheese on oatcake*

malted drinks – *milk with vanilla extract*

milk shakes – *unsweetened yoghurt shakes*

ice-cream – *unsweetened frozen yoghurt*

sorbet/water ice – *chilled oranges*

Condiments

jam – *Marmite/Bovril*

syrups – *honey*

tomato ketchup – *home-made tomato purée*

dessert toppings – *cream*

prepared sauces (check label for sugar content) – *home-made sauces*

colas/fizzy drinks – *mineral water*

cordials/squashes – *mineral water*

SAMPLE SUBSTITUTION PROGRAMME

* Items marked with an asterisk are given in greater detail in the Snack Substitutes and Recipes sections (pp. 313, 324).

MONDAY

Breakfast

Normal 2 slices wholemeal toast with butter and marmalade; sugary cereal with milk; sweetened orange juice; coffee with milk and sugar

Includes these Stop Foods Marmalade, sugary cereal, sweetened orange juice, sugar

Substitute 2 slices wholemeal toast with butter and Bovril; branflakes with yoghurt, no sugar; mineral water; black coffee

Elevenses

Normal I biscuit; coffee with milk and sugar

Stop Biscuit, sugar

Substitute *I plain oatcake; coffee with milk

Lunch

Normal Sausage roll and salad; chocolate bar; cola; coffee with milk and sugar

Stop Chocolate bar, cola, sugar

Substitute Bowl of soup; sausage roll and salad; *banana and cream; sparkling mineral water; coffee with milk

Afternoon tea

Normal Piece of cake; cup of tea with sugar

Stop Cake, sugar

Substitute *2 rice cakes spread with flavoured diet fromage frais; cup of tea without sugar

Dinner

Normal Prawn cocktail with 2 slices brown bread; pasta in tomato sauce with courgettes; ice-cream; chocolates

Stop Ice-cream, chocolates

Substitute Prawn cocktail with 2 slices brown bread; *pasta in tomato sauce with courgettes; *plain yoghurt mashed with frozen raspberries; cheese and crispbread

TUESDAY

Breakfast

Normal 2 chocolate biscuits; fresh orange juice; coffee with milk and sugar

Stop Biscuits, sugar

Substitute I soft-boiled egg with 2 slices brown bread and butter; fresh orange juice; coffee with milk, no sugar

Elevenses

Normal American-style cookie; coffee with milk and sugar

Stop Cookie, sugar

Substitute Cheese and tomato sandwich; coffee with milk, no sugar

Lunch

Normal Chicken salad; individual portion fruit trifle; glass wine; chocolate bar; coffee with milk and sugar

Stop Trifle, chocolate bar, sugar

Substitute Chicken salad; chips or baked potato; unsweetened yoghurt with nuts or fruit; wine; sparkling mineral water; banana; coffee with milk, no sugar

Afternoon tea

Normal Small bar of chocolate; tea, no sugar

Stop Chocolate

Substitute *Banana and Ryvita sandwich

Dinner

Normal Packet of potato crisps; sausages; baked beans; 2 slices toast; flavoured jelly; 2 glasses wine; coffee; 1 chocolate truffle

Stop Baked beans, jelly, truffle

Substitute Packet of potato crisps; sausages; *home-cooked mixed pulses in fresh tomato sauce; 2 slices toast; unsweetened muesli with milk and cream; wine; coffee; tangerine

WEDNESDAY

Breakfast

Normal Cereal with milk; pancake with maple syrup; fresh squeezed orange juice; coffee

Stop Cereal, maple syrup

Substitute Oatflakes with milk and chopped banana; pancake with butter and honey; fresh squeezed orange juice; coffee

Elevenses

Normal Shortcake biscuit; coffee

Stop Shortcake biscuit

Substitute *Rice cake spread with flavoured cottage cheese; coffee

Lunch

Normal Scotch egg salad; chocolate bar; cola; chocolate dessert; coffee with milk and sugar

Stop Chocolate bar, cola, chocolate dessert, sugar

Substitute Scotch egg salad; 2 slices bread and butter; sparkling mineral water; apple and cheese; coffee with milk, no sugar

Afternoon tea

Normal Snack bar; tea, no sugar

Stop Snack bar

Substitute *Oatcake; tea

Dinner

Normal Bowl of soup; grilled lamb chop; spinach; mashed potato; tinned tomato; tinned fruit salad; coffee without sugar

Stop Tinned fruit salad

Substitute Bowl of soup; grilled lamb chop; spinach; mashed potato; fresh fruit salad and cream; coffee without sugar

THURSDAY

Breakfast

Normal 2 chocolate biscuits; cola; coffee with milk and sugar

Stop Biscuits, cola, sugar

Substitute 2 rashers of bacon and 1 fried egg on a thick slice of soda bread; fresh orange juice; coffee, no sugar

Elevenses

Normal Chocolate digestive biscuit; coffee, no sugar

Stop Biscuit

Substitute *2 Ryvitas spread with honey and flavoured cottage cheese; coffee

Lunch

Normal Baked potato with cheese; salad; chocolate gâteau; coffee; Coca Cola

Stop Chocolate gâteau, Coca Cola

Substitute Baked potato with cheese; salad; *mashed banana with yoghurt and crumbled oatcake; coffee; Diet Coke

Afternoon tea

Normal Egg sandwich; tea

Stop None

Substitute None

Dinner

Normal Taramasalata with brown bread; commercially prepared cod and salmon fish pie; spinach; grilled tomatoes; ice-cream; 2 glasses wine; coffee; after-dinner mint

Stop Commercially prepared meal (if ingredients list includes sugar, if not no need to substitute); ice-cream; mint

Substitute Taramasalata with brown bread; if fish pie contains sugar, then *home-made fish pie, otherwise don't worry; *frozen yoghurt; 2 glasses wine; kiwi fruit

FRIDAY

Breakfast

Normal Toast with jam; coffee with milk and sugar

Stop Jam, sugar

Substitute Toast with butter and Marmite; fresh orange juice; black coffee

Elevenses

Normal Doughnut; coffee, no sugar

Stop Doughnut

Substitute Banana sandwich; coffee

Lunch

Normal Pork pie with chutney; tomato salad; sponge pudding with treacle; 2 glasses wine; coffee; chocolate bar

Stop Sponge pudding with treacle, chocolate bar

Substitute Pork pie with chutney; tomato salad; mashed banana and cream; cheese and crispbread; 2 glasses wine; coffee

Afternoon tea

Normal Ginger biscuit; tea

Stop Ginger biscuit

Substitute *Ryvita and flavoured cottage cheese; tea

Dinner

Normal 3 measures spirit; Chinese take-away; 2 glasses wine; china tea; mint

Stop Any sweet or sweet and sour Chinese dishes, mint

Substitute 3 measures spirit (if you must); Chinese take-away without dishes like sweet and sour pork or crispy beef; 2 glasses wine; china tea; orange quarters

SATURDAY

Breakfast

Normal 1 slice toast with jam; coffee

Stop Jam

Substitute 1 slice toast with butter and Marmite; coffee; sparkling mineral water

Elevenses

Normal Doughnut; coffee

Stop Doughnut

Substitute Tuna sandwich; coffee

Lunch

Normal Pub lunch of bread, cheese, chutney, salad; gâteau; ½ pint shandy

Stop Gâteau

Substitute Pub lunch of bread, cheese, chutney, salad, chips; fruit salad; ½ pint shandy

Afternoon tea

Normal Cake; tea

Stop Cake

Substitute Honey and cottage cheese sandwiches made with soda bread; tea

Dinner

Normal 2 measures spirit; avocado filled with prawns; steak; peas; baked potato; grilled tomatoes and mushrooms; ice-cream; 3 glasses wine

Stop Ice-cream

Substitute 2 measures spirit (it is Saturday after all); avocado filled with prawns; steak; peas; baked potato; grilled tomatoes and mushrooms; fresh fruit salad; sparkling mineral water

SUNDAY

Breakfast

Normal Danish pastry; sugar-frosted cereal with milk; hot chocolate drink

Stop Danish pastry, sugar-frosted cereal, hot chocolate drink

Substitute Bacon; grilled continental sausage slices; toasted soda bread; grilled tomatoes; fresh squeezed orange juice; milky coffee

Elevenses

Normal Chocolate bar; coffee with milk and sugar

Stop Chocolate bar, sugar

Substitute Quartered orange; coffee, no sugar

Lunch

Normal 2 measures spirit; roast pork; mashed potato; cabbage; peas; gravy; apple pie with cream; coffee

Stop Apple pie

Substitute 2 measures spirit; roast pork; mashed potato; cabbage; peas; gravy; *stewed fruit (oranges, bananas, peeled sliced apples) with cream and a garnish of crumbled oatcake; coffee

Afternoon tea

Normal Biscuit; tea

Stop Biscuit

Substitute I slice toasted soda bread with honey; tea

Dinner

Normal Spanish omelette; salad; bread; cheese; celery; 2 glasses wine; chocolates

Stop Chocolates

Substitute Spanish omelette; salad; bread; cheese; celery; 2 glasses wine; mixed nuts

---

NEW THINKING ON EATING DISORDERS

What are eating disorders?

A person is said to have an eating disorder when their eating pattern is so chaotic and irregular that it jeopardises health and happiness. The three main disorders are: anorexia – refusal to eat; bulimia – binge-eating followed by purging; compulsive eating – continual repetitive overeating. Generally, by the time the eating disorder has reached this clinical level the sufferer is beyond the point of self-help. Thus the occasional binge, followed by guilt and a successful resolution not to repeat the episode for a month, would not constitute an eating disorder. Nor would occasional loss of appetite.

What causes eating disorders?

There are many different theories about the cause of eating disorders, and the three main types – anorexia, bulimia and compulsive eating – seem to have different causes. There is considerable evidence to show that chemical imbalances within the brain may predispose someone to be at risk of developing an eating disorder, but environmental factors are probably at work too. So far there has been little research into whether eating disorders can be genetically inherited, and in time this may be revealed as a factor.

Who gets eating disorders?

Anybody can develop an eating disorder, and it is not in fact a modern phenomenon. The 'green sickness' of young girls in the Middle Ages and later 'the vapours', are now thought to be early names for eating disorders. Most people think that eating disorders are confined to the wealthy West, but this is not necessarily the case. Eating disorders are more difficult to diagnose in those whose diet is already chaotic due to difficulties in obtaining food, but deliberate fasting, purging and compulsive eating of certain foods exist all over the world.

However, the epidemiology of eating disorders does show certain groups to be more at risk than others. Adolescent girls from wealthy Western cultures form the most readily identifiable and highly researched group. But the idea that eating disorders almost exclusively affect the middle classes has now been discredited. Current thinking is that they are spread among all socio-economic groups, but the middle classes tend to report and seek help for eating disorders more than other groups.

Though largely afflicting women, men too suffer all three forms of eating disorders.

Can these disorders be cured?

All three main types of eating disorder can be cured, but external help (preferably professional) is almost always needed. Due to recent work on hypoglycaemia and on endorphins, there is now considerable knowledge about how to break the vicious binge-purge syndrome of bulimia. Less good headway has been made in the fields of compulsive eating and of anorexia. Compulsive eating has only relatively recently been regarded as a discreet eating disorder, qualitatively different from habitual overeating.

The picture with anorexia is complicated by prejudice and the overtones of neurosis which the nineteenth-century term anorexia nervosa carried. Most anorexics still report that the treatment they are offered is ineffective and unsympathetic, but the situation is gradually improving.

If I am fat or I eat a lot does it mean I have a disorder?
Neither anorexics nor bulimics present as overfat. Eating a lot does not in itself mean a disorder. A healthy appetite should always be applauded. But where eating is associated with compulsive and obsessional behaviour, some borderline disorder might be suspected.

ANOREXIA

Some Possible Causes

The main contributing factor to anorexia is currently regarded to be psychological. The aetiology seems to be that the sufferer has a basically obsessive compulsive personality (extreme perfectionism, self-discipline, etc.) to which is added an above average capacity for self-denial. Very often this is coupled with family problems that give rise to an urgent need for the sufferer to suppress her emotions and emotional needs.

The sufferer's drive is to find some way to express and enact her painful emotions and need for help. The preoccupation of our society with idealised women's bodies makes a preoccupation with thinness and achieving a 'perfect' body a convenient peg on to which to project the sufferer's unhappiness. In the early stages this is often unwittingly reinforced by those who praise the sufferer for her slim figure and ability to diet.

An additional problem for young girls seems to be today's pressures to conform to conflicting stereotypes. It is now not only acceptable but positively encouraged for young women to have careers. An intelligent and sensitive young woman may find herself under a great deal of pressure to be a high achiever. At the same time she finds pressures on her socially to be attractive and outgoing and to mix readily with other members of her peer group. Yet it can be extremely hard to achieve conformity in both areas. And when it comes to her early encounters with the opposite sex she may find a great deal of reserve and suspicion among adolescent boys about her high-achieving image.

Because of their pre-existing perfectionist tendencies, girls at risk of anorexia are likely to try to conform on every front, which can trigger the initial diet. The 'success' of the initial diet encourages the sufferer to continue the activity. Even at this stage full anorexia has not taken hold. Eventually though, the original rational and emotional subconscious 'reasons' for dieting are subsumed by the need for the diet itself. The impulse to fast, and thus exercise a control over emotional needs and even life events, becomes the dominant driving force and anorexia is established.

Negative Therapies

Much treatment of anorexics has been misguided and ineffective. Methods have included forced eating; emphasis on achieving weight gains; behaviour modification.

Logically it is hard to see how anyone can believe in forced eating as an approach capable of long-term success. The old saying is that you can lead a horse to water but you can't make it drink. Forced eating may keep the severe anorexic alive long enough to undergo other therapies, but it can never be an answer in itself unless you are prepared to force-feed an anorexic for the rest of her life.

Weight gain goals are again at best a temporary measure to control symptoms. If they are unaccompanied by other therapy, then as soon as the anorexic obtains her weight goal and leaves medical care she will simply embark on another fast.

Behaviour modification – where the sufferer is punished for not eating until her aversion to the therapy supposedly outweighs her aversion to eating – has worryingly Dickensian workhouse overtones, but can be helpful if it is combined with other more positive approaches.

Positive Therapies

Psychopharmacy (medication for psychological disorder) is among the newer approaches, with the controversial medication Prozac achieving some good results.

Psychotherapy (counselling for psychological disorder) is effective, but requires long-term commitment on all sides. However, it is almost certainly the most beneficial approach, with the most lasting results. Therapies may include analysis or behavioural therapy or hypnotherapy.

Vitamin therapy, where sufferers take a range of supplements – especially zinc and B group vitamins – has shown some success in alleviating appetite disorder, but there is little hard evidence at the moment.

Associated problems

Compulsive exercising; agoraphobia (fear of interaction with other humans); mood swings.

Diets and the Anorexic

Conventional slimming diets are in fact much less related to anorexia than we might think. However, unscrupulous slimming advice may provide ammunition to an anorexic. None of the eating plans in this book includes any element of fasting or dietary imbalance which might contribute to anorexia.

Recommended eating plans:
- Borderline anorexic – Low-sugar Eating Plan (p. 97)
- Anorexic – Vegetarian/Special Requirements Eating Plan (pp. 294, 279) with professional help and counselling.
- Recovering anorexic – Low-processing Eating Plan (p. 152).

BULIMIA

Some Possible Causes

The binge-purge syndrome of bulimia was originally seen as no more than a variant of anorexia. At one time they both shared the suffix 'nervosa'. It is now becoming apparent that bulimia is quite distinct from anorexia.

Bingeing and purging has been practised by humans at least since the days of the Roman Empire and has gone through periods of being almost an accepted phenomenon. In the bulimic, though, it is taken to the level of an addiction. This is one of the primary differences between bulimia and anorexia: while anorexia is a compulsion, bulimia is now seen to be an addiction.

The bulimic becomes addicted to the cycle of vast intake followed by an immense sense of release and relief on vomiting. Anyone who has ever had gastric flu knows just how much better you feel for a minute or so after vomiting. The bulimic obtains the same 'high' from her vomiting and becomes addicted to the sensation. It is believed that this is because the act of emptying the stomach by retching signals the brain to release endorphins, the body's natural opiates.

An acute bulimic may go through as many as 10 or 15 episodes in a day. But unlike anorexia, the effects of the condition are not visible. The bulimic will go to great pains to hide her habit and her body weight will probably remain stable. This means that bulimia is not an expressive illness. Like anorexics, bulimics may have great problems with their emotions, but very often they come from a background which seeks to hide and deny any acknowledgement of unwanted emotions or family problems.

The emphasis is to appear normal, to disguise distress. Bulimics are likely to face the same pressures to conform to high career and social achievement as anorexics, but usually they appear externally to succeed outstandingly on these levels. Bulimics tend to be copers and binge-purging is their secret escape.

Psychologists believe that the act of vomiting contains a metaphor of the bulimic ridding herself forcibly of all the unwanted emotions she has been forced to repress and bury within herself. There also seems to be a strong link between bulimia and the hypoglycaemia syndrome we discuss on p. 100.

Another undoubted feature of bulimics is that they are able to vomit voluntarily more readily than the average. Many bulimics in fact discover bingeing and purging during ordinary post- and pre-diet binges.

Conventional slimming diets do therefore seem to play a much greater role in triggering bulimia than in anorexia.

Treatment

Because bulimia is difficult to spot and less immediately life-threatening than anorexia (though still dangerous to health), bulimics tend not to receive much treatment at all. Bulimics who seek treatment voluntarily usually obtain some kind of counselling therapy.

Associated problems

Self-mutilation (self-cutting, self-bruising); mood swings; destructive relationships; occasionally alcoholism and other addictions; in extreme cases bulimia can cause oesophagal ulcers and tooth damage.

Course of Action

Follow the Low-sugar Eating Plan (p. 97) closely and obtain therapy (check addresses on p. 334 and speak to your family doctor).

COMPULSIVE EATING

The symptoms of compulsive eating disorder are very similar to those of congenital and chronic obesity – that is, constant overfat and repeated failed diet attempts coupled with habitual overeating.

The main problem for the compulsive overeater is chronic low self-esteem. They must maintain an unacceptable level of fat on their bodies in order to have something on which to project their feelings of low self-worth and self-hatred. If they allowed themselves to become thin they would have to face their lack of self-esteem more directly.

Compulsive eaters find their repeated diet attempts a useful distraction. Starting a diet offers an illusory promise of a better life, and failing to achieve it confirms their existing low opinion of themselves. Eating may also act as a metaphor for feeding the emotions, so that the on/off diet syndrome expresses the conflict between needing to receive emotional input and being unworthy to receive it.

As in all cases of eating disorder, professional psychological help is the best long-term answer. Again Prozac may be a helpful medication in raising self-esteem levels. Because compulsive eating has something in common with congenital obesity, it would also be a good idea to read the ideas on pp. 53–72.

Treatment
Therapy; congenital obesity eating plan (p.53).

WHAT NEXT?

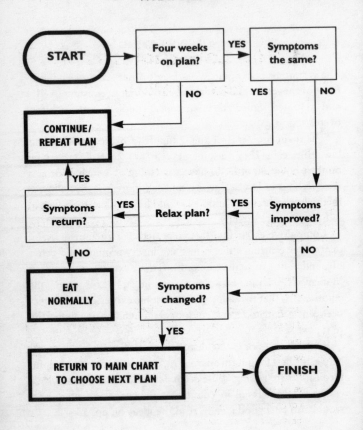

4. The Low-cholesterol Eating Plan

LOW-CHOLESTEROL PLAN CHECK CHART

Before you start the Low-cholesterol Eating Plan, fill in the check chart by ticking any Yes answers to double-check you have chosen the most appropriate eating plan.

1. I am male. ☐
2. I know I have a cholesterol problem. ☐
3. My family has a history of heart/arterial disease. ☐
4. I find it very difficult to stay calm and cool in difficult situations. ☐
5. Certain foods seem to upset me more than others. ☐
6. I have very sensitive skin. ☐
7. I have high blood pressure. ☐
8. I have never liked physical activity. ☐
9. I am often tense and anxious. ☐
10. I've never cared much about what I eat. ☐

Ticks KEY

0–3 The Low-cholesterol Eating Plan is not appropriate for you.

4–8 Your life-style and health would be much improved by the Low-cholesterol Eating Plan.

9–10 This eating plan may still be the best one for you to follow but you should also consider the Low-processing and Low-allergen Eating Plans (pp. 152, 259). If you answered Yes to 6, you could again

consider looking at the Low-allergen Eating Plan (p. 259), since skin
sensitivity is often associated with allergy.

IMPORTANT: If you answered Yes to both 2 and 7, make sure you
have regular medical checks – vital if you also answered Yes to 3.
Your family doctor will have advice for you. Also note the British
Heart Foundation address (p. 334).

WELCOME TO THE LOW-CHOLESTEROL PLAN

The word cholesterol is bandied about so much these days that
even experts who ought to know better are beginning to take it
for granted that they know what it means. In fact it is now being
used so inaccurately and in such a muddled way that I think it is
time we got absolutely straight what cholesterol is and why this
eating plan is appropriate for you.

Cholesterol is an almost insoluble sterol found in nearly all
animal tissues. Many people assume cholesterol and fat are the
same thing. In fact sterol is not a fat but a waxy, sticky cell
substance. Cholesterol in itself is not a bad thing. It is naturally
present in our bodies, where it plays a role in insulating the nerve
sheaths and is involved in hormonal processes.

There are two main kinds of cholesterol in our bodies: HDL
(high density lipoprotein) and LDL (low density lipoprotein).
Another variant has also been found recently, known as VLDL
(very low density lipoprotein).

Over the last couple of decades a great deal of research into
the Western world's high rates of heart disease and arteriosclerosis has pointed towards a link between heart disease and a high
level of LDL in the blood.

Now first of all, let's get it straight that this is what is
scientifically known as an epidemiological observation, not an
experimental result supporting a hypothesis. In other words the
theory is drawn from the research, rather than the research being

carried out to test the theory. However, the statistical evidence is so overwhelming that Western governments and health bodies like the British Heart Foundation are convinced that high levels of LDL cholesterol in the blood are not only linked with heart disease, but are a risk factor pointing towards later contraction of the disease. Reducing levels of blood LDL cholesterol through medication or diet is believed to reduce the risk of coronary disease by as much as 25 per cent.

So far it all seems perfectly straightforward. Eat less cholesterol; have less cholesterol in your body; stay free of heart disease.

If only life were that simple. The first stumbling block arose about a decade ago when doctors and scientists began to differentiate between dietary cholesterol and blood cholesterol. Blood cholesterol is exactly what it sounds – the cholesterol that is present in your own blood. But dietary cholesterol is cholesterol you take in with the food you eat (not to put too fine a point on it, it was some other unfortunate animal's blood cholesterol).

It had been thought that the more dietary cholesterol you ate the more blood cholesterol you would have. It sounded logical enough, but more and more studies began to turn up anomalies. It was found that many people with a high cholesterol diet (like obsessive egg-eaters) actually had very low blood cholesterol levels. Whereas lots of very thin people with low cholesterol diets had high blood cholesterol levels.

Biologists pointed out that the body can both excrete dietary cholesterol and manufacture its own blood cholesterol from other ingredients, so in all likelihood the actual level of dietary cholesterol eaten probably has very little effect on levels of blood cholesterol.

It is also widely known that the 'fight or flight' reaction caused by stress can stimulate the production of blood cholesterol. In this reaction the stomach is drained of blood and adrenalin pumped into the blood to enrich it for a sudden burst of energy. If the sudden burst of energy never comes, the enriched blood is liable to lay down cholesterol. The moral of this is that the next time you feel like hitting your boss, you should do so. It will be good for your health, if not your career.

Despite these blips, the basic statistical link between high levels of blood cholesterol and heart disease was still too strong to ignore, so scientists began to look more closely at the relationship. This time animal fats generally rather than specific dietary cholesterols were pinpointed as important in the cholesterol/coronary link. Today the accepted belief is that eating too much animal fat is a factor in heart disease, and that blood cholesterol levels are involved in the process.

Recently even this advice has become controversial. Some new studies have shown that those whose blood cholesterol levels are successfully lowered through diet or medication have the same prognosis of death as before. But instead of dying of heart disease they tend to die from vehicle accidents or suicide. Personally I think these new studies have been over-emphasised. Certainly they do not carry the authoritative weight of evidence of the government's low-fat campaign.

So how does all this relate to you, the low-cholesterol eating planner? Here are the facts from research as it stands today, without all the media hype:

- By reducing the amount of LDL cholesterol in your blood you stand a very good chance of reducing your risk of heart/artery disease.
- If you already have heart/artery disease reducing the amount of LDL cholesterol in your blood is an important element of treatment.
- Heart/artery disease is partly hereditary, so if you have a genetic risk then aiming to keep your blood LDL cholesterol levels low could be a good insurance policy.

- A low-fat diet is believed to help lower blood cholesterol levels.
- Do not confuse dietary cholesterol with blood cholesterol. A high intake of dietary cholesterol does not always result in high blood cholesterol.
- If you are at risk of heart/artery disease it is safer to reduce both dietary fat and dietary cholesterol.
- Diet is not the only element to play a role in heart/artery disease. Other factors include obesity, smoking, stress, fitness, genetics and temperament.

CHOLESTEROL TYPES CHECK CHART

HDL (good cholesterol)	LDL (bad cholesterol)	VLDL (bad cholesterol)
High Density Lipoprotein, involved in metabolic processes, not a health threat, manufactured by the body.	Low Density Lipoprotein, believed to contribute to arterial disease, manufactured by the body and possibly ingested in the diet. Excess assumed to be due to dietary causes and stress.	Very Low Density Lipoprotein, recently identified, may be shown to have the more significant role in arterial disease.

HOW IT WORKS

The Low-cholesterol Eating Plan has been designed taking into account all the current medical thinking, and aiming for the safest possible compromise between the opposing sides in the controversy. The great advantage of this eating plan, like all the plans throughout this book, is that it is aimed at a specific group of people. By going through the diagnosis chart and checking your findings at the beginning of the chapter, you have discovered the eating plan that is likely to be of most benefit to you personally. Unlike government guidelines, which give everybody the same advice regardless, this eating plan is only for people who do have or are likely to develop a cholesterol problem.

I always find it immensely irritating to be given irrelevant advice. In the case of the cholesterol controversy, advice that is simply off-target may also be dangerous. Those who are sceptical about the case against cholesterol will almost certainly have chosen a different eating plan, but those to whom it strikes home as an important and relevant area are on the right plan for them. Before you start the plan read the notes below about stress, since I think it is important to work on both fronts at once. After the advice on stress comes a step-by-step guide to this eating plan. Just follow the guide to how to stop and substitute foods in your diet and you'll find it plain sailing.

STRESS

I suspect that we will soon be presented with evidence that stress plays at least as important a part in heart disease as does diet. Today there is a great deal of advice available on stress reduction. You can get it from books, magazines, your family doctor, even your workplace. Pursue these avenues and bear in mind the following tips:

- Be aware of the areas of your life which might be stressing you.
- Don't punish yourself or be guilty about feeling stressed.
- Learn the difference between situations you can do something about and those you can't affect.
- No matter how tired, always spend some time relaxing before going to sleep – perhaps reading or taking a bath.

- Take up an outdoor leisure pursuit (walking, golf, fishing, etc.).
- Envisage the worst case scenario in order to defuse your worries about a particular situation.
- Don't rely repeatedly on alcohol, food, medication, etc. to distract you from your stressed feelings.
- Seek help from professionals, family and friends.
- Keep smiling and breathe slowly, using your diaphragm.
- Don't shut yourself off from social life.

STEP-BY-STEP GUIDE TO THE LOW-CHOLESTEROL PLAN

1 Read all sections of the diet carefully.

2 Learn what the stop foods are and why you must stop eating them.

3 Get familiar with all the substitutes and where to buy them.

4 Go through the week-long sample eating programme and work out how it will fit into your lifestyle.

5 If you are at all uncertain you can decide to follow the sample eating programme exactly for a week until you get the hang of things.

6 Learn how to make the snack substitutes.

7 Make a copy of the glance guide to stop and substitute foods.

8 Take the glance guide shopping with you to make sure you are stocking up on the right foods.

9 Remember that any food not mentioned as a stop food can be eaten whenever you like.

10 Note which drinks are to be stopped.

11 Eat plenty of fresh vegetables, these are not stop foods.

12 Follow the diet for about 2 months before reviewing your symptoms and deciding whether to continue on it, change to another diet, or return to normal eating.

STOP, THINK, SUBSTITUTE

Which foods should I stop eating and what should I substitute?

Complex Carbohydrate Group

According to government health watchdogs in Britain and the United States, altering the diet of someone at risk of heart disease or having a high blood cholesterol so that it contains about 50 per cent complex carbohydrates and around 25 per cent fats substantially improves that person's health prognosis.

Modern Western diets tend to have more than 30 per cent fat in them (perhaps up to 40 per cent) and as little as 30 per cent complex carbohydrates. Countries where the incidence of heart disease is low tend to be those where the diet is high in complex carbohydrates. Current nutritional thinking is that this is not a coincidence (but nobody has proved that conclusively, as there are too few controls to perform the experiment successfully).

The recommendation therefore is to increase the number and quantity of complex carbohydrates you eat. So make sure you have plenty of bread, pasta, rice, root vegetables, beans/pulses and cereals.

There has recently been considerable publicity about the role of oats in decreasing blood cholesterol levels. Oats are high in soluble fibre. The theory is that this glutinous material somehow causes potential cholesterol-forming fats to be stuck to it and rapidly excreted from the system, since fibre is indigestible.

However, some doubts have now been cast over the quality of controls established in some of the research experimentation. Be that as it may, oats are an excellent complex carbohydrate, rich in nutrients as well as soluble fibre, so it makes sense to use oat-based products frequently (see below for their use as a substitute food).

Another advantage of complex carbohydrates is that they are good nutritional value for calories and they have a role in decreasing appetite for other, less healthy, foods.

- **Stop:** White bread, white rice.

- **Substitute:** Variety grain bread, brown and wild rice.

Refined Carbohydrate Group

While complex carbohydrates are nutritional good news for the low-cholesterol planner, refined carbohydrates are the reverse. A refined carbohydrate is basically a complex carbohydrate which has been processed so that only sugar remains and all the other components of complex carbohydrate (fibre, water, minerals, vitamins, trace elements, some protein) have been discarded.

Nutritionists advise that we should reduce the amount of sugar we eat, largely because it is calorie-dense and nutritionally poor value for calories. This makes obvious sense for those on the Low-calorie, Low-sugar, and Low-processing Eating Plans, but the low-cholesterol eating planner might legitimately inquire why this should be applied to him. After all, sugar is completely free of animal fat and cholesterol.

There are several reasons why the low-cholesterol planner must be careful about refined carbohydrates:

- According to the BMA (British Medical Association), an excess of refined carbohydrates in the diet may contribute to increased cholesterol levels under certain circumstances (e.g. times of stress, chronic exhaustion).
- Raised blood cholesterol and the diseases linked with it are usually found present in a complex of ill-health factors. These factors include obesity and diabetes, both of which are linked with excess intake of refined carbohydrates.
- Preferred food products in the West where refined carbohydrates are among the ingredients are almost always

presented in combination with fats, e.g. biscuits, where
sugar is presented with butter.

- **Stop**: Sugar-laden foods including sugary breakfast cereals,
  biscuits, commercial puddings and cakes, confectionery;
  sweet fatty foods like croissants, doughnuts, crackers,
  pâtisserie.

- **Substitute**: Plain oat-based cereals and porridge; variety,
  mixed grain and continental breads; oatcakes, crispbreads
  and bread with honey, cottage cheese and/or low-fat
  fromage frais, fruit; dried fruit.

Protein Group

Though cholesterol is rarely found in plants, it is present in
animal tissues – from which we in the West obtain most of our
protein. Though there is still considerable debate about the role
played by high animal protein intake in raised blood cholesterol
levels, it is better to be safe than sorry. So if you know you have a
cholesterol or artery/cardiac problem, it makes sense not to add a
possible risk factor by continuing to eat sources rich in dietary
cholesterol.

- **Stop**: Fatty meats; dark red meats; fried/roast meat and
  fish; commercial meat products including sausages, pâté,
  pork pies, Scotch eggs, convenience meals; fatty nuts
  (peanuts and Brazils); fish roe (including caviar and
  taramasalata); egg yolks; seafood.

- **Substitute**: Grilled, casseroled or stir-fried lean and white
  meats; grilled or poached fish; beans, pulses, etc.; low-fat
  cottage cheese.

Vegetable and Fruit Group

Plenty of fruit and vegetables will be great allies in maintaining a
low-cholesterol plan. Not only are they good nutritional value

for calories, they also satisfy the appetite and many contain the same sort of soluble fibre as oats. Prepared imaginatively, vegetables can be an exciting element in the diet – check out the Vegetarian Eating Plan (p. 294) for some ideas.

- **Stop**: Deep-fried vegetables (chips, etc.); roast vegetables; deep fried fruit fritters; avocado pears.

- **Substitute**: Stir-fried, raw or steamed vegetables; fresh fruit; aubergines (same mouth appeal as avocado without the fat).

Dairy and Fats Group

Despite some dissenting voices, the current consensus of opinion is that saturated animal fats are doing most to contribute to the raised levels of artery and heart disease in the Western world. The assumption being made is that high consumption of saturated animal fat leads to high levels of blood cholesterol and increased risk of atheromas (the narrowing of the coronary artery by a fatty deposit). These atheromas are the main factor in coronary artery disease.

Time and again leading health bodies (including NACNE and the British Heart Foundation) have put forward the following formula: high animal fat leads to high cholesterol leads to heart disease. This superficially logical theory is the accepted conventional thinking about cardiac/arterial disease. I do not dispute it. Nor if I were a scientist would I wholeheartedly endorse it. Yes, it is logical, but it still remains very largely an assumption. Not enough genuinely controlled experiment has been done to prove the theory incontrovertibly.

The message to hold on to, though, is that although the theory may not quite stand up to rigorous scientific inquiry – *in practice it works well enough.*

So you are advised to switch from animal to vegetable fats if you are a low-cholesterol eating planner.

- **Stop**: Full cream milk; cream; hard and cream cheeses; butter; rice pudding; chocolates; full cream milk shakes; saturated cooking oils; lard; dripping; suet.

- **Substitute**: Skimmed milk; fromage frais/low-fat yoghurt; low-fat spread; porridge with skimmed milk; bananas; yoghurt shakes; olive or polyunsaturated oil; polyunsaturated margarine.

Condiments

Any sauces, flavourings and seasonings containing a high proportion of animal fat or dietary cholesterol should be avoided.

- **Stop**: Mayonnaise; peanut butter; commercial savoury nibbles.

- **Substitute**: Low-calorie salad cream; honey/Marmite/ Bovril; raw vegetable sticks.

Eating Out and Take-away

Apply common sense to your eating out and take-aways. When eating out these days there are nearly always good low-fat and low-cholesterol options on the menu. Some restaurants even put a special asterisk against their low-fat options so that you can spot them easily. So many businessmen have been told to reduce fat to cut their cholesterol that restaurants would be very foolish indeed not to provide them with something to eat. Ask the waiter to recommend a suitable dish.

If the restaurant is unenlightened you can still do fine. Choose a fruit or salad based starter or soup. For the main course choose a grilled lean white meat or fish with plenty of vegetables, salad, and baked, boiled or mashed potatoes. Dessert can be fruit, jelly, meringue (but not cream).

Some forms of take-away are fattier than others. Fried fish and chips are off limits.

Indian take-away can be pretty fatty – even the breads are often fried. Choose chapatti rather than nan or poppadom. Choose tandoor-roast dishes rather than pasandas and biryanis. Basically, if it looks greasy, it's fatty.

Greek take-away is usually chargrilled and free from fatty sauces. The oil used in cooking should also be olive oil. If it's not olive oil they're not real Greeks. Choose a grilled lamb or chicken kebab in pitta bread with salad. Dolmades (stuffed vine leaves) are great but avoid taramasalata (have tzatsiki instead) and the heavy dishes like moussaka and stifado.

Chinese take-away is a minefield, as every Chinese chef cooks differently. Minimise the damage by opting for stir-fried rather than deep-fried dishes; fish, chicken and vegetables rather than duck and meat; boiled rice rather than fried rice.

If you've ever eaten a real Italian pizza you'll realise what a travesty the ones you get in Britain are. Instead of being a crisp nutritious mix of complex carbohydrates and vegetables with a little garnish of cheese or meat, they are mammoth, fatty, gooey dumplings with the healthy tomato purée more or less non-existent and the fatty cheese topping swollen out of proportion. Enough said. Enough said too about burgers and shakes. Burgers are OK if they really are made of excellent beef well-grilled over a flame and served in a granary bun without cheese or butter. The shakes you can stand your toddler upright in are never OK, ever, for anyone.

AT-A-GLANCE GUIDE TO
STOP AND SUBSTITUTE FOODS

Stop – *Substitute*

Complex Carbohydrate Food Group

white bread – *brown bread*
white rice – *brown rice*

Refined Carbohydrate Food Group

sugared breakfast cereals – *plain oat-based cereals, unsweetened muesli*
croissants – *hot granary rolls*
biscuits – *oatcakes*
savoury crackers – *Ryvita*
commercial puddings – *diet fromage frais*
commercial cakes – *fruit*
doughnuts – *oatcakes with honey*
pâtisserie – *soda bread with honey and cottage cheese*
confectionery – *fruit, dried fruit*

Protein Food Group

roast meats – *grilled, casseroled or stir-fried lean meats and fish*
sausages – *grilled fish fingers/fish cakes*
pâté – *cottage cheese/vegetarian spreads*
commercial pies and meals – *fish pie, home-made stews*
bacon – *grilled continental hams*
fried fish – *grilled or poached fish*
fried or breadcrumbed meats – *meats with a potato topping*
peanuts – *raisins*
Brazil nuts – *sultanas*
fish roe (including caviar) – *diced salmon (marinaded or smoked)*
taramasalata – *tzatsiki (cucumber blended with yoghurt)*
egg yolks – *egg whites or, for cooking, culinary egg substitute*

Vegetable and Fruit Food Group

chips – *crisp stir-fried carrot and parsnip sticks*
roast potatoes – *baked potatoes*
potato crisps – *nuts (not roasted or salted), raisins*
avocado pears – *aubergine*

Dairy Food Group

full cream milk – *skimmed milk*
cream – *fromage frais, yoghurt*
hard cheeses – *Edam, Gouda, low fat cheese*
cream cheese – *cottage cheese*
rice pudding – *porridge with skimmed milk*
milk shakes – *yoghurt shakes*
chocolates – *bananas*

Fats Group

butter – *low fat spread*
saturated cooking oils – *olive oil or polyunsaturated oil*

fats – *polyunsaturated margarine*
dripping/lard/suet – *polyunsaturated margarine*

Condiments

salt – *herbs/low-salt*
mayonnaise – *low-calorie salad cream*
peanut butter – *Marmite/Bovril*
commercial savoury nibbles – *raw vegetable sticks*

SAMPLE SUBSTITUTION PROGRAMME

* Items marked with an asterisk are given in greater detail in the Snack Substitutes and Recipes sections (pp. 313, 324).

MONDAY

Breakfast

Normal 2 slices wholemeal toast with butter and marmalade; cereal with milk; sweetened orange juice; coffee with whole milk and sugar
Includes these Stop Foods Butter, cereal, sweetened orange juice, whole milk
Substitute 2 slices wholemeal toast with polyunsaturated margarine and marmalade; pure oatflakes (no salt or sugar, check pack) with skimmed milk; fresh squeezed orange juice; coffee with skimmed milk (sugar if desired)

Elevenses

Normal 1 biscuit; coffee with milk and sugar

Stop Biscuit, whole milk

Substitute 1 plain oatcake; coffee with skimmed milk

Lunch

Normal Bowl of soup; sausage roll and salad; apple; 1 glass wine

Stop Sausage roll

Substitute Bowl of soup; 2 granary rolls and salad; apple; 1 glass wine

Afternoon tea

Normal Piece of cake; cup of tea with whole milk, no sugar

Stop Cake, whole milk

Substitute *2 rice cakes spread with flavoured diet fromage frais; cup of tea with skimmed milk

Dinner

Normal Prawn cocktail with 2 slices brown bread and butter; commercial spaghetti bolognaise with courgettes; ice-cream

Stop Prawn cocktail, butter, commercial spaghetti bolognaise, ice-cream

Substitute Melon with 2 slices brown bread and polyunsaturated margarine; *risotto with tomatoes and herbs; courgettes; *plain yoghurt mashed with frozen raspberries

TUESDAY

Breakfast

Normal Soft-boiled egg with 2 slices bread and butter; fresh orange juice; coffee

Stop Egg yolk, butter

Substitute *Scrambled egg whites with skimmed milk and herbs; 2 slices granary bread and polyunsaturated margarine; fresh orange juice; black coffee

Elevenses

Normal American-style cookie; black coffee

Stop Cookie

Substitute Orange; coffee

Lunch

Normal Fried chicken limb in breadcrumbs; chips; peas; individual portion fruit trifle; glass wine; coffee

Stop Fried chicken, chips, trifle

Substitute Plain grilled chicken limb; baked potato with polyunsaturated margarine; peas; fruit salad with yoghurt; glass wine (but preferably sparkling mineral water); coffee with skimmed milk

Afternoon tea

Normal Small bar of chocolate; tea

Stop Chocolate

Substitute *Banana and Ryvita sandwich

Dinner

Normal Packet of potato crisps; sausages; baked beans; 2 slices toast; flavoured jelly; 2 glasses wine; coffee; 1 chocolate truffle

Stop Potato crisps, sausages, truffle

Substitute Handful of unsalted nuts and raisins; *fresh vegetable risotto; baked beans; 2 slices toast with polyunsaturated margarine; jelly; 2 glasses wine (but preferably sparkling mineral water); black coffee; tangerine

WEDNESDAY

Breakfast

Normal Cereal with milk; pancake with maple syrup; fresh squeezed orange juice; coffee

Stop Cereal, whole milk, pancake, maple syrup

Substitute Oatflakes with skimmed milk and chopped banana; wholemeal toast with polyunsaturated margarine and honey; fresh squeezed orange juice; black coffee

Elevenses

Normal Shortcake biscuit; black coffee

Stop Shortcake biscuit

Substitute *Rice cake spread with flavoured cottage cheese; coffee

Lunch

Normal Scotch egg salad; 2 slices brown bread; apple; wine; coffee

Stop Scotch egg

Substitute Fresh cold poached salmon with large continental salad; 2 slices brown bread with polyunsaturated margarine; apple; mineral water; coffee

Afternoon tea

Normal Snack bar; tea

Stop Snack bar

Substitute *Oatcake; tea

Dinner

Normal Bowl of soup; grilled lamb chop; spinach; mashed potato; tinned tomato; fresh unsugared fruit salad; coffee

Stop None

Substitute None

THURSDAY

Breakfast

Normal 2 rashers of bacon and 1 fried egg on toast; fresh orange juice; coffee

Stop Bacon, fried egg

Substitute Large bowl of porridge made with skimmed milk, no salt added, but brown sugar permitted; 2 slices brown toast with honey and polyunsaturated margarine; fresh orange juice; coffee with skimmed milk

Elevenses

Normal Chocolate digestive biscuit; coffee

Stop Biscuit

Substitute *2 Ryvitas spread with honey and flavoured cottage cheese; black coffee

Lunch

Normal Baked potato with cheese; salad; chocolate gâteau; coffee; Coca Cola

Stop Cheese, chocolate gâteau

Substitute Baked potato with cottage cheese and grated raw carrot; salad; *mashed banana with yoghurt and crumbled oatcake; coffee; Diet Coke

Afternoon tea

Normal Egg sandwich; tea

Stop Egg

Substitute 2 slices Ryvita sandwiched round sliced tomato with polyunsaturated margarine; tea with skimmed milk

Dinner

Normal Taramasalata with brown bread; commercially prepared cod and salmon fish pie; spinach; grilled tomatoes; ice-cream; 2 glasses wine; coffee; after-dinner mint

Stop Taramasalata, commercially prepared meal (check fat content), ice-cream

Substitute *Tzatsiki with plain bread roll; *home-made fish pie (using olive oil for frying; skimmed milk for sauce and mashed potato for topping); spinach; grilled tomatoes; *frozen yoghurt; 2 glasses wine; after-dinner mint

FRIDAY

Breakfast

Normal Toast with butter and jam; coffee

Stop Butter

Substitute Toast with polyunsaturated margarine and honey; fresh orange juice; coffee

Elevenses

Normal Apple; coffee with whole milk

Stop Whole milk

Substitute Apple; coffee with skimmed milk

Lunch

Normal Pork pie with chutney; tomato salad; 2 glasses wine; coffee
Stop Pork pie
Substitute Rice salad; tomato salad; 2 glasses wine (but preferably fresh orange juice); coffee

Afternoon tea

Normal Ginger biscuit; tea
Stop Ginger biscuit
Substitute *Ryvita and flavoured cottage cheese; tea

Dinner

Normal 3 measures spirit; Chinese take-away; 2 glasses wine; coffee; mint
Stop Any deep-fried Chinese dishes
Substitute 3 measures spirit (if you must); Chinese take-away without deep-fried dishes; 2 glasses wine; coffee; mint

SATURDAY

Breakfast

Normal Sausage sandwich; coffee
Stop Sausage sandwich
Substitute Orange segmented and garnished with roasted almonds; coffee; sparkling mineral water

Elevenses

Normal Doughnut; coffee
Stop Doughnut
Substitute Fruit tart; coffee. While not ideal, a fruit tart is a good weekend compromise!

Lunch

Normal Pub lunch of bread, cheese, chutney, salad, chips; ½ pint shandy
Stop Cheese, chips
Substitute Pub lunch of gammon with pineapple; salad; baked potato with cottage cheese or polyunsaturated margarine; ½ pint shandy

Afternoon tea

Normal Cake; tea

Stop Cake

Substitute Honey and cottage cheese sandwiches made with soda bread; tea

Dinner

Normal 2 measures spirit; avocado filled with prawns; fried steak; peas; baked potato; grilled tomatoes and mushrooms; ice-cream; 3 glasses wine

Stop Avocado filled with prawns, fried steak, ice-cream

Substitute 2 measures spirit (it is Saturday, after all); *mushroom vinaigrette; grilled sole; peas; baked potato; grilled tomatoes and mushrooms; fresh fruit salad; 3 glasses wine

SUNDAY

Breakfast

Normal Bacon; sausage; fried bread; grilled tomatoes; orange juice; coffee

Stop Bacon, sausage, fried bread

Substitute Porridge with skimmed milk and brown sugar; 2 slices toast with polyunsaturated margarine and honey; fresh squeezed orange juice; coffee

No elevenses today

Lunch

Normal 2 measures spirit; roast pork; roast potatoes; cabbage; peas; gravy; apple pie with cream; coffee

Stop Roast pork; roast potatoes; gravy; cream

Substitute 2 measures spirit; *chicken and cucumber casserole; mashed potato; cabbage; peas; pan juice reduction; apple pie with yoghurt; coffee

Afternoon tea

Normal Biscuit; tea

Stop Biscuit

Substitute I hot bread roll with honey, no butter; tea

Dinner

Normal Spanish omelette; salad; bread; cheese; celery; 2 glasses wine

Stop Omelette, cheese

Substitute *Fresh vegetable ratatouille; salad; bread; cottage cheese; celery; 2 glasses wine

WHAT NEXT?

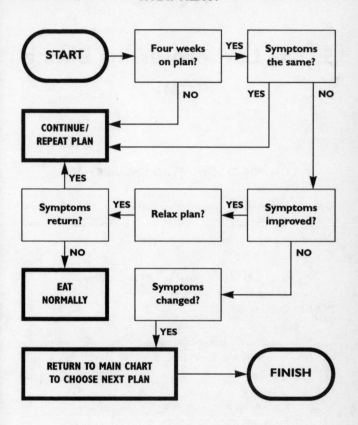

5. The Low-processing Eating Plan

LOW-PROCESSING PLAN CHECK CHART

Before you start the Low-processing Eating Plan, fill in the check chart by ticking any Yes answers to double-check you have chosen the most appropriate eating plan.

1. The hours I work make it difficult for me to eat healthily. ☐
2. I very often eat out or buy take-away. ☐
3. I don't eat very much. ☐
4. I've never cared much about what I eat. ☐
5. My hair and skin are in poor condition. ☐
6. I frequently suffer from constipation. ☐
7. My clothes feel too small for me. ☐
8. I get a lot of colds. ☐
9. Friends notice how thirsty I always am. ☐
10. Even though I'm slim my stomach gets very bloated. ☐

Ticks KEY

0–3 The Low-processing Eating Plan is not ideal for you at present. Use the chart to assess exactly what your most pressing symptom is. It may be that you can revert to the Low-processing Eating Plan after dealing with more urgent problems.

4–8 A low-processing diet will bring you up to a good nutritional state and make you feel much healthier. If you answered Yes to 4, it is unlikely that you have been paying enough attention to the nutritional quality of what you eat. If you answered Yes to 8, there may be an indication that poor diet has lowered your immune system.

9–10 Check through the flow chart carefully before choosing your eating plan. Low-processing may be right, but you should also consider the Anti-candida Eating Plan (p. 228).

IMPORTANT: Answering Yes to 9 is one of the symptoms of diabetes. Check the Special Requirements Eating Plan (p. 279).

WELCOME TO THE LOW-PROCESSING EATING PLAN

Humans first started preserving and processing their foods for the very best of reasons – to make them digestible, hygienic, healthy and pleasant to eat. Very soon – you may be surprised to learn that it was many hundreds of years ago – commercial interests began to enter the area of food and there has been a downhill slide more or less ever since, leading us to the present day when the processing of food is a politically hot issue.

First of all, it is very important not to get this out of proportion. Without preserving and processing our food, life as we enjoy it today would not be possible. Cooking meat is a form of processing it, and one which has made the difference between us and every other omnivore/carnivore on the planet. The cooking of meat aids and speeds digestion, so that instead of lying around digesting for 16 hours a day like the big cats, humans can get on with inventing the wheel and so forth.

Preserving food is equally vital, and centuries ago we discovered ways of preserving by drying, smoking, salting, cooking in sugar, and soaking in vinegar or oil. The industrial revolution, when millions of people began to live together in cities without ready access to a food supply, would not have been possible had we not known how to preserve food long enough to transport it. So it is quite ridiculous to say that the processing and preserving of food is bad in and of itself.

Before the industrial revolution most people relied largely on food they had grown or raised themselves. Extras were bought at market, but only after a very close inspection, and the consumer expected to be cheated through short measure, doctoring and bulking of food, and for the food not to be as fresh as advertised.

With the growth of the large cities after the industrial revolution, a high percentage of the population became urban and were unable to grow or raise their own food. They had to rely on what the market traders and the burgeoning new class of food retailers brought into the city. The quality of this food, particularly for the poorer classes, was low. Contamination of food, both accidental and deliberate, was rampant. Flour was bulked and whitened with powdered chalk; milk was watered to make it go further.

The great Victorian social reformers campaigned so successfully for government regulations on food standards and safety that by the mid-twentieth century the standard of bought food was probably better than it had ever been in the history of Britain. During the Second World War, food rationing and government dietary advice and propaganda ensured a brief period of very healthy eating. For a short time in our history food was readily available that was processed in such a way as to free it from possible contamination, yet was not over-processed or over-preserved. After the war, however, the scene was set for tastes to swing the other way again, and palates jaded by wartime rationing welcomed the 1950s invention of highly processed novelty foods. By the 1970s, though, it was recognised that foods were once more in danger of contamination – this time through over-processing.

The health food boom was born, and shops selling loose lentils, stone-milled flour, herb tea and so forth sprouted (almost literally in some cases) on every high street. Trading standards officers had a terrible time, and I can well remember in the early 80s reporting a whole series of health food disasters. A woman died when her herbal tea was contaminated with deadly nightshade. There was an outbreak of violent food poisoning from a mouldy walnut yoghurt. Packets of dried mushrooms were found to include fibres from poisonous fungi. Dried apricots turned out to contain a carcinogenic chemical. And legions of people broke teeth on bits of gravel and stone in pulses and flour.

There was even a group of home bakers who began hallucinating because the 'organic' flour they were using contained the fungus ergotamine. This was particularly interesting for historians, because ergot was the scourge of the Middle Ages. An evil-looking little black rice-grain-shaped fungus that hides in wheat ears, the ergot was widespread and frequently contaminated bread. It is a well-known hallucinogenic, and some historians believe it had quite a lot to do with the high incidence of miracles such as walking statues and angelic visions during medieval times!

Oddly enough, the health food boom was proof of just what good quality our food has become in the twentieth century. To be able to take food hygiene so much for granted that you would risk buying it from unmonitored, non-factory sources shows a confidence in bought food that would not have been shared by any of our predecessors. Unprocessed and unpreserved food is by no means necessarily healthy food. In fact it can be quite dangerous.

Today both types of food – 'faddy' and often under-processed health foods; and over-processed convenience foods – exist side by side. If we can draw a healthy compromise between the two, the stage could be set for another period of safe, healthy eating.

Types of Convenience Foods

Food type	Examples	Processing elements
Instant (both sweet and savoury)	Powdered soups, powdered desserts, drink mixes, shake mixes, whips, cake mixes, sauces, gravies	Sugars including malt glucose etc., salts including monosodium glutamate, flavouring both natural and artificial, flour, emulsifier, anti-caking agents, colouring
Sweet	Biscuits, cakes, breads, jams, spreads	Sugar, fat, flour, lactose, powdered egg, cocoa, colouring, flavouring, anti-oxidant
Savoury	Meat pies, sausages, cold cuts, burgers, pork pies	Mechanically recovered meat, salts, sugars, fat, water, breadcrumbs, flavourings, colourings, anti-oxidants
Long shelf-life	Juices, some dairy, cakes, biscuits, confectionery, tinned foods, dried foods	Heat treatment for liquids, colourants, preservatives, etc.
Novelty	Breakfast cereals, 'invented foods', confectionery, sweet but savoury foods, potato crisps and other packet snacks	Sugar, salts, fats, anti-oxidants, colourings, flavourings
Convenience	Pre-prepared and frozen ready meals, etc.	Freezing, bulking and glazing through water addition, emulsifiers

| Junk | Take-away foods | Multi-phase cooking and re-heating, artificial bulkers, sugar, fat, salt, colouring, flavouring |

Types of Additive

Type	Used for	Why necessary
Cosmetic	Improving colour, taste, smell and texture of food	To give the illusion of quality and palatability in second-rate foodstuffs
Preservatives	To prevent oxidation and other forms of decay	Important for hygiene in many nutritious but short-lived foods, also necessary to give commercially desirable long shelf-life and storage
Processing aids	Raising agents, emulsifiers, anti-caking agents, glazing agents, bleaches and improvers	To make food ingredients behave in an organically unnatural way in order to obtain a commercially viable novelty food

For perhaps 20 years we ate and enjoyed highly processed, mass-marketed novelty foods without a second thought. Then the evidence of carcinogens and allergens in artificial additives began to appear. Today in the 90s we can see that the backlash of the health food boom was an over-reaction, but the fact remains that there is a health risk in having a diet that contains too great a proportion of highly processed, low-nutritive-content, novelty 'junk' foods.

There is plenty you can do to eat a safe and satisfying diet without becoming a health food nut. As usual, the key is moderation. Ignore the hysterical stories you will read in the media. Yes, risks do exist, but for those who eat a generally balanced diet with a high proportion of fresh foods, correctly cooked, they are not a major concern.

But how many of us today do eat that wonderfully balanced diet? When the pressures of your life take you to the stage where you are almost constantly eating out, taking-away or browsing on junk food, it is time to start thinking seriously about how you can improve the quality of your diet. Since you have chosen the Low-processing Eating Plan, you are almost certainly already at this stage. Take hope, it's not too late in the day to save the situation!

Just a few simple alterations in your eating can make you feel healthier, slimmer and more energetic. It has nothing to do with calorie-counting. It's just a matter of learning how not to be so dependent on modern processed foods, without turning it into an obsession.

The following table shows the concerns nutritionists have voiced about highly processed foods. Some, like food poisoning, are now a major cause for concern, while others demonstrate an ultra-cautious approach to food risks.

CURRENT CONCERNS OVER HIGHLY PROCESSED FOODS

Widespread Concerns			
Food fault	**Explanation**	**Health concern**	**Risk foods**
Bacterial infection	Salmonella, campylobacter, listeriosis	Food poisoning, birth defects	Pre-prepared chiller cabinet foods, factory farmed meats
High sugar content	Main ingredient = refined carbohydrate	Obesity, hypoglycaemia	Hard sell non-staple treat foods

Allergenic	Containing additives (usually artificial) to which eater is allergic	Asthma, eczema, migraine, etc.	'Instant' foods, long-shelf-life dry foods, novelty foods
High fat content	More than 30% saturated animal fat	Obesity, arterial disease, possible breast cancer	Junk food, prepared meat products, cakes and biscuits
Carcinogenic	Containing additive or nitrite residue, carrying cancer risk	Various cancers	Some 'diet' products, especially diet soft drinks, nitrogen residue foods
Low nutritive value	Insufficient vitamins, protein, etc.	Borderline malnutrition, deficiency symptoms	Children's novelty foods, junk food, pre-prepared convenience meals

Rarer Health Concerns

Diseased (very rare)	May be contaminated by or carry an animal disease, e.g. BSE (bovine spongiform encephelomyelitis)	Birth defects, illness, brain damage (even death)	Junk food, prepared meat products (especially those containing MRM – mechanically recovered meat), factory farmed meat products

High salt	Sodium group minerals	Raised blood pressure, fluid retention, electrolytic imbalances	Junk food, long-shelf-life pre-prepared foods
Pesticide residue	Trace contaminants of chemical insect, weed and fungus killers	Cancers, allergies, birth defects	Factory farmed fruit and vegetables
Hormone residue	Trace residue of hormones used to promote lactation, fatten, etc.	Human hormonal imbalances, fertility and potency problems	Factory farmed meats
Antibiotic residue	Build up of antibiotics used to control spread of disease	Immune system imbalances, candida, allergy	Intensively reared animals
Nitrate concentration	Built up from fertiliser leaching and forms into nitrites and N-nitroso	Cancers	Intensively reared animals, intensively grown cereals, contaminated water table (especially East Anglia)
Chemical content	Chemical additives used in preserving, colouring, processing, etc.	Allergic reactions, hyperactivity in children, possible cancer risks	Novelty foods, junk food

HOW IT WORKS

I'm not asking you to become a crank or spend all your time cooking, or to look different from your friends. The Low-processing Eating Plan is all about finding food that is convenient and pleasant to eat, but that doesn't carry the drawbacks of junk food. Fortunately there are loads of good foods that naturally come in convenient portions and packing and don't require a lot of preparation. It is even possible to eat out and to eat take-away without exposing yourself to lots of undesirable processing elements.

When you are eating in, one of the first steps is to ensure that your ingredients are the best possible. Even though they are a little more expensive, organically grown fruit and vegetables are not only healthier but taste a lot better.

Check to make sure you really are buying free range eggs (if they don't say 'free range' in exactly those words it means they aren't). Try to get your meat from a supplier of non-intensively farmed animals. This is becoming much easier today. Even some national supermarkets have started selling 'open farmed' meat from animals (including pigs) guaranteed to be reared outdoors. This is a step forward, but for the best meat ever, find a rare-breeds farm that is selling surplus stock. To put it bluntly, it will have lived happy, died happy and will eat happy. There are some addresses on p. 336 to help you.

Now read on – the Step-by-step Guide will take you through exactly what you need to do to start the Low-processing Eating Plan.

STEP-BY-STEP GUIDE TO THE LOW-PROCESSING EATING PLAN

1   Read all sections of the diet carefully.

2   Learn what the stop foods are and why you must stop them.

3   Get familiar with all the substitutes and where to buy them.

4   Go through the week-long sample eating programme and work out how it will fit into your lifestyle.

5   If you are at all uncertain, you can decide to follow the sample eating programme exactly for a week until you get the hang of things.

6   Learn how to make the snack substitutes.

7   Make a copy of the glance guide to stop and substitute foods.

8   Take the glance guide shopping with you to make sure you are stocking up on the right foods.

9   Remember that any food not mentioned as a stop food can be eaten whenever you like.

10 Note which drinks are to be stopped.

11 Eat plenty of fresh vegetables, these are not stop foods.

12 Follow the diet for at least 2 months before reviewing your symptoms and deciding whether to continue on it, change to another diet, or return to normal eating.

STOP, THINK, SUBSTITUTE

Which foods should I stop eating and what should I substitute?

Complex Carbohydrate Group

Complex carbohydrates are the starchy foods derived from plant matter that provide the staple energy source in the human diet. The complex carbohydrates include grains such as wheat, rye, oats, maize, barley (from which breads and pastas are made) and rice (a grain also comparatively high in protein). Apart from these well-known complex carbohydrates, other sources include root vegetables (such as potatoes) and the bean/pulse family.

During the 60s and 70s, wholegrain versions of the complex carbohydrates became very fashionable. The obsession with home-made bread and lentil stew eventually became so ridiculous that in the 80s there was a backlash. Experts pointed out that some degree of processing and preservation of food was vital to prevent its contamination and deterioration and to render it more digestible. Indeed, many cases of contamination and decay in 'wholefoods' were reported, and without doubt much of the so-called 'health food' eaten was more or less indigestible or unpleasant to eat.

Nevertheless, over-processing of complex carbohydrates to present a more commercially acceptable and marketable food does deplete the high nutritional value originally present. Along with energy calories, most complex carbohydrates also comprise fibre, water, vitamins, minerals, trace elements and some protein. Many of these components (especially fibre and minerals) are contained in the part of the food that is discarded during processing.

In some products an effort is made to replace these components artificially (e.g. flour improver in white bread), which seems quite ridiculous. The best compromise is to stop eating highly processed complex carbohydrates where the substitutes available are safe, palatable (often more so) and healthy.

- **Stop:** White bread; frozen bread; dried/tinned pasta/spaghetti.

- **Substitute:** Wholemeal and continental breads; fresh bread (if time try making your own); fresh pastas.

Refined Carbohydrate Group

The refined carbohydrate group represents a more extreme version of the situation outlined above. All the foods human beings eat are processed in some way. From earliest times man has threshed wheat to separate the grain from the stalk, and then further processed it by winnowing to separate the germ from the chaff (bran), thus making it a more readily available source of energy. Later forms of processing were concerned with preserving foodstuffs in order to be able to store excess for times of famine.

The process of creating a refined carbohydrate combined these two aims with absolute success. By processing complex carbohydrate sources to the point where only one element was left and all the others discarded, man created the most readily available possible source of energy, which also virtually never deteriorated.

The wonder product is of course sugar, our name for refined carbohydrate. Very little refined carbohydrate exists in nature. Honey is the most obvious example, where the refining work is performed by bees.

However, the simple fact that sugar is produced by human processing is not what makes it unsuitable for the low-processing eating planner. The problem with sugar is largely the way mankind currently uses it. Instead of using it as a simple preservative (as in jam) or as a basic sweet treat (as in confectionery), we now use sugar to make palatable and long-lasting a whole range of foods that would not otherwise be so.

In the making of many meat products, for example, sugar is used in combination with other seasonings (and often manufactured chemicals) in order to turn mechanically recovered tissue (gristle, offal, bone scraping, gut lining, etc.) into food that is not just palatable but actually desirable.

Many of our favourite dessert mixes are nothing more than bulking agents (cellulose or starch-gel) combined with emulsifiers (often artificially manufactured), seasonings and a large amount of sugar.

So while refined carbohydrate, sugar, as such is not a problem for the low-processing planner, the highly processed products in which it so often appears should be limited and substituted wherever possible.

- **Stop**: Commercial cakes, biscuits, doughnuts, puddings, desserts, cake mixes; sugary breakfast cereals; snack bars; pre-prepared pasta dishes; anything with a long shelf-life (check sell-by date); bought pizza; pot noodles and instant food mixes.

- **Substitute**: Home-made cakes, biscuits and desserts (if no time, do without); breads and crispbreads with topping; home-made fruit and tea breads (if time); muesli/porridge; sandwiches; fresh pastas in home-made sauces; home-made snacks such as soup or baked potatoes.

Protein Group

Many modern highly processed foods are extremely difficult to classify nutritionally, particularly protein-based convenience food products. Perhaps the supreme example of this is the familiar sausage, which could appear in almost every food group except beverages! A sausage contains breadcrumbs, so it can be placed in the complex carbohydrate group. It usually contains sugar, so it can also be placed in the refined carbohydrate group. It certainly contains some meat so it fits into the protein category as well. Often a sprinkling of parsley or diced vegetables may be among the ingredients, which puts it in the vegetable group. As is obvious when it is cooked, the sausage also contains a large amount of fat, so it can be placed in that group as well.

This ought to make sausages a super-food. Surely they are a balanced meal in a skin! Yet we know perfectly well that sausages are junk food. This is because modern processing allows almost every single individual ingredient of the sausage to be presented in its most debased form. Instead of fresh whole-grain bread, dried white bread powder is used. Sugar is already a nutritionally debased carbohydrate. The meat used is not fresh organic open-farmed muscle tissue. It is in fact the most disgusting looking meat-slurry I have ever seen, mechanically scraped from joint sockets, organ linings and otherwise unpalatable (and even unmentionable) parts of the animal. Herbal or plant seasoning comes in the form of a dried powder. Large quantities of animal fat are used to bind the whole lot together and make it tasty, along with salt and sometimes artificial chemical seasonings (such as monosodium glutamate).

A home-made sausage (and you can get them in some restaurants and from enlightened organic suppliers) might be a very different thing. The ideal sausage would be soft brown breadcrumbs mixed with chopped parsley and tomato, then stirred into a reasonable quantity of fine minced fillet steak or fish, and the whole bound together with olive oil and egg yolk. I think you would find sugar or artificial seasoning would be unnecessary.

So for the low-processing planner there is nothing wrong with protein in itself, only with its modern day debased presentation.

- **Stop**: Convenience food; junk food; sausages; ham; factory-farmed meat; pre-packed long-shelf-life meat; deep frozen meat; battery eggs; ready meals; tinned meat and fish products.

- **Substitute**: Sandwiches/restaurant food; fish and chips for junk food; organic meats (fresh, from a good butcher or supplier); free range eggs; cold meat and salad for ready meals.

Vegetable and Fruit Group

Time and again for the low-processing planner the problem lies not with a particular food group, but with the way it is today presented for consumption. Thus raw vegetables made into salads and coleslaws and eaten fresh are wonderful, but the pre-prepared coleslaws and pot salads you can buy now have a comparatively long shelf-life (which entails the addition of a preservative, often sugar) and a complex set of ingredients (often including fat) which alter the nutritional composition of the original dish. The coleslaw you prepare at home from fresh vegetables, fruits and home-made dressing and eat immediately is nutritionally light years removed from the one residing in your fridge after you chose it from the supermarket chiller cabinet last week.

Other aspects of processing also decrease and alter the nutritional state of fruit and vegetables. Chemical residues and waxing may add toxins. Long periods of chilling involved in transport or poor farming practices may reduce nutritional value – as well as making the food less appetising.

- **Stop**: Prepared pots of salads and coleslaw; tinned vegetables; tinned fruit; out of season, long distance imported (outside EC) and waxed fruit; potato crisps; commercially prepared vegetable meals.

- **Substitute**: Fresh, local and seasonal produce as far as possible; organic fruit and vegetables, not over-stored or over-cooked.

Dairy and Fats Group

Fortunately recent nutritional thinking is rehabilitating such natural, wholesome products as butter and whole milk. Providing you are healthy, allergy-free, not overfat, not morally opposed to animal cultivation, and do not have risk factors predisposing towards certain degenerative diseases, there is no reason why you should not enjoy a glass of creamy milk and a piece of toast smothered in butter.

And here's a shock. The vast majority of people living in Britain today fall into this category.

I know. If you've lived here (as opposed to Mars) at any time during the last decade you will find this virtually impossible to believe. But it's true. And if you are one of the majority, then for heaven's sake don't allow yourself to be brow-beaten by the media into one food panic after another.

Highly processed alternatives to dairy and fat products are widespread, but they are not as tasty and satisfying as the natural originals and because they have not been tested over as long a period of time may carry mild health risks of their own. So if you don't have to use them, why bother?

- **Stop**: Commercially prepared milk shakes and dairy drinks; long-life dairy products; ready whipped cream and toppings; low-fat spreads; margarine; cooking oil; ready-mixed dips.

- **Substitute**: Dairy drinks made at home by whizzing yoghurt and fruit juice in a blender; fresh milk; double cream; butter/dripping; virgin olive oil; home-made dips.

Condiments

The condiment group is the one that has been least affected by the trend towards 'healthy' eating over the last couple of decades. Highly processed, multi-ingredient condiments are largely a product of this century. In the past, food was seasoned during cooking, or presented in a sauce, rather than having that seasoning or sauce added by the eater at the table.

High-quality food has never needed much enhancement by seasoning or sauces. That is why British food is plain compared with so many other cuisines. Historically Britain has always been a good place for farming (particularly animal cultivation), and therefore high-quality ingredients were readily available. Unlike many European countries, even British peasants generally had access to food of a quality that made clever cooking unnecessary.

During the industrial revolution this situation changed. In Victorian cities the poorer classes had little access to good fresh food because they had no opportunity to cultivate it themselves. It is no coincidence that this is about the period when pre-prepared condiments first began to appear commercially.

The commercial condiment makes palatable highly processed food that would otherwise be unacceptable. Have a hot dog without ketchup or mustard; try a burger without mayo or chilli, and you'll see what I mean.

- **Stop**: Sauce mixes; snacks/nibbles; 'novelty' foods; topping mixes; commercial pickles.

- **Substitute**: Pan juice reductions; olives/nuts; raw vegetables; double cream; home-made pickles/nuts/olives.

Beverages

The particular beverages the low-processing planner decides to substitute will largely depend on how hard a line you are taking on processing. Avoiding soft canned drinks, certainly those with artificial colourings and flavourings, is fairly obvious. Some though are virtually no more than sugar and carbonated water, and while it may horrify you to realise that that is what you are enjoying, that may not be a reason to avoid them.

Thornier is the question of tea and coffee. Tea especially is no more highly processed than flour, and indeed was once regarded as a healthy brew. The 'PG' in PG Tips, for example, comes from the phrase 'pro-gastration', invented by the manufacturers to stress the supposed beneficial effects of tea on the digestion.

I suggest that you begin your Low-processing Eating Plan by substituting all the stop foods until you feel stable enough to make your own choices. There are compromises – for example, you might choose to have only fresh as opposed to instant coffee.

- **Stop**: Coffee; tea; colas/fizzy drinks; concentrate fruit drinks and squashes.

- **Substitute**: Milk; bouillon (a stock drink); spiced hot fresh orange juice; hot lemon juice and honey; mineral water; tomato juice; unsweetened fruit juices.

Eating Out and Take-away

Because the ingredients of a particular dish cannot be guaranteed, eating out or take-away is something of a minefield for the low-processing planner, unless you are wealthy. There are lots and lots of wonderful restaurants in Britain where you can get fresh, low-processed food prepared simply and deliciously, but unfortunately they tend to be rather expensive.

Wherever you eat, however, there will usually be dishes with very simple recipes that are not likely to contain highly processed ingredients – a basic fish or steak dish with plain vegetables is usually the safest bet.

With take-away you will just have to use your common sense. From what you have read you will know that the junk food which forms most take-away is not advisable on your plan. That said, there are some take-aways which do not rely on highly processed food, mainly from the ethnic cuisines.

A good Indian take-away, for example, may well be high in fat and calories but is often made with wonderfully healthy basic ingredients. The Chinese, on the other hand, have a tendency to chuck monosodium glutamate into every dish.

AT-A-GLANCE GUIDE TO STOP AND SUBSTITUTE FOODS

Stop – *Substitute*

Complex Carbohydrate Food Group

white bread – *wholemeal bread/ continental breads*
frozen bread – *fresh bread*
dried/tinned pasta/spaghetti – *fresh pasta*

Refined Carbohydrate Food Group

cakes – *home-made jam tarts, etc.*
biscuits – *Ryvita and topping*
doughnuts – *bread with honey and cream cheese*
commercial puddings/desserts – *home-made apple pie*
cake mixes – *home-made fruit breads*
breakfast cereals – *muesli/porridge*

snack bars – *sandwiches*
pre-prepared pasta dishes – *fresh pasta and home-made sauce*
anything with a long shelf-life – *check sell-by dates*
pizza – *stuffed baked potato/risotto*
pot noodle – *soup*
instant food mixes – *something fresh!*

Protein Food Group

convenience food – *sandwiches/ restaurant food*
junk food – *fish and chips*
sausages – *spare ribs*
ham – *cold beef*
factory farmed meat – *organic meat*
pre-packed meat – *butcher's meat*
frozen meat – *fresh meat*
battery eggs – *free range eggs*
ready meals – *cold meat and salad*
tinned meat products – *fresh meat*

Vegetable and Fruit Food Group

prepared salad/coleslaw pots – *fresh raw salads*

tinned vegetables – *frozen vegetables*

tinned fruit – *fresh fruit*

out of season fruit – *local seasonal fruit*

long-distance imported vegetables – *frozen/local fresh vegetables*

waxed fruits – *organically grown fruits*

potato crisps – *olives*

commercial vegetable meals – *fresh raw salad*

Dairy Food Group

milk shakes – *yoghurt blended with fruit*

long-life products – *fresh milk*

ready whipped cream – *fresh double cream*

low-fat spreads – *butter*

margarine – *butter/dripping*

cooking oil – *virgin olive oil*

ready-mixed dips – *home-made dips*

concentrate fruit drinks and juices – *fresh fruit juice*

Condiments

sauce mixes – *pan juice reductions*

snacks/nibbles – *olives/nuts*

'novelty' foods – *raw vegetables*

topping mixes – *double cream*

commercial pickles – *home-made pickles/nuts/olives*

SAMPLE SUBSTITUTION PROGRAMME

* Items marked with an asterisk are given in greater detail in the Snack Substitutes and Recipes sections (pp. 313, 324).

MONDAY

Breakfast

Normal 2 slices white toast with butter and marmalade; sugary cereal with milk; sweetened orange juice; coffee with milk and sugar

Includes these Stop Foods White bread, sugary cereal, sweetened orange juice, coffee

Substitute 2 slices Hovis bread toast with butter and marmalade; pure oatflakes with milk; fresh squeezed orange juice; *hot lemon juice with honey (or 1 cup coffee from morning allowance of two cups)

Elevenses

Normal 1 biscuit; coffee (from morning allowance)
Stop Biscuit
Substitute 1 orange; coffee

Lunch

Normal Baked potato; grated cheese; salad; Coca Cola
Stop Coca Cola
Substitute Baked potato; grated cheese; salad; mineral water

Afternoon tea

Normal Piece of cake; cup of tea without sugar (from afternoon allowance of 1 cup of tea)
Stop Cake
Substitute *2 rice cakes spread with flavoured diet fromage frais; cup of tea

Dinner

Normal Prawn cocktail with 2 slices brown bread; pasta in tomato sauce with courgettes; ice-cream
Stop Ice-cream
Substitute Prawn cocktail with 2 slices brown bread; *fresh pasta in tomato sauce with courgettes; *plain yoghurt mashed with frozen raspberries

TUESDAY

Breakfast

Normal Soft-boiled egg with 2 slices bread and butter; fresh orange juice; coffee from allowance
Stop None
Substitute None

Elevenses

Normal American-style cookie; coffee from allowance
Stop Cookie
Substitute Orange; coffee

Lunch

Normal Fried chicken limb in breadcrumbs; chips; peas; individual portion fruit trifle; 1 glass wine; coffee
Stop Chicken in breadcrumbs, trifle, coffee (excess of allowance)
Substitute Plain grilled chicken limb; chips; peas; fruit salad with yoghurt; 1 glass wine; *hot lemon juice with honey

Afternoon tea

Normal Small bar of chocolate; tea from allowance
Stop Chocolate
Substitute *Banana and Ryvita sandwich

Dinner

Normal Packet of potato crisps; sausages; baked beans; 2 slices toast; flavoured jelly; 2 glasses wine; coffee; 1 chocolate truffle
Stop Potato crisps, sausages, baked beans, coffee (excess of allowance), truffle
Substitute Handful of olives and unsalted nuts; grilled spare ribs marinated in tomato juice, honey, sherry and lemon juice; *home cooked mixed pulses in fresh tomato sauce; 2 slices toast; jelly; wine; *Piermont; tangerine

WEDNESDAY

Breakfast

Normal Novelty breakfast cereal with milk; pancake with maple-flavoured syrup; fresh squeezed orange juice; coffee
Stop Cereal, maple-flavoured syrup
Substitute Oatflakes with milk and chopped banana; pancake with real maple syrup; fresh squeezed orange juice; coffee

Elevenses

Normal Shortcake biscuit; coffee

Stop Shortcake biscuit

Substitute *Rice cake spread with flavoured cottage cheese; coffee

Lunch

Normal Scotch egg salad; 2 slices brown bread; apple; wine; coffee

Stop Scotch egg, coffee in excess of allowance

Substitute Egg mayonnaise; large continental salad; 2 slices brown bread; apple; wine; mineral water

Afternoon tea

Normal Snack bar; tea

Stop Snack bar

Substitute *Oatcake; tea

Dinner

Normal Bowl of soup; grilled lamb chop; spinach; mashed potato; tinned tomato; fresh fruit salad; coffee

Stop Tinned tomato, coffee in excess of allowance

Substitute Bowl of soup; grilled lamb chop; spinach; mashed potato; diced and stewed tomato; fresh fruit salad; *hot milk flavoured with vanilla essence

THURSDAY

Breakfast

Normal 2 rashers of pre-packed bacon and 1 fried egg on toast; fresh orange juice; coffee

Stop Pre-packed bacon

Substitute 2 rashers of loose bacon (preferably farmed in the open) and 1 fried egg on toast; fresh orange juice; coffee

Elevenses

Normal American cookie; coffee

Stop American cookie, coffee

Substitute Bread and honey; *hot spiced orange juice

Lunch

Normal Baked potato with cheese; salad; chocolate gâteau; coffee; Coca Cola
Stop Chocolate gâteau, Coca Cola, coffee in excess of allowance
Substitute Baked potato with cheese; salad; *mashed banana with yoghurt and crumbled oatcake; mineral water; *hot lemon juice with honey

Afternoon tea

Normal Egg sandwich; tea
Stop None
Substitute None

Dinner

Normal Taramasalata with brown bread; commercially prepared cod and salmon fish pie; spinach; grilled tomatoes; ice-cream; 2 glasses wine; coffee; after-dinner mint
Stop Commercially prepared meal, ice-cream, coffee in excess of allowance
Substitute Taramasalata with brown bread; *home-made fish pie; *frozen yoghurt; 2 glasses wine; *Piermont; after-dinner mint

FRIDAY

Breakfast

Normal Toast with jam; coffee
Stop None
Substitute None

Elevenses

Normal Apple; coffee
Stop None
Substitute None

Lunch

Normal Pork pie with chutney; tomato salad; 2 glasses wine; coffee
Stop Pork pie, chutney, coffee in excess of allowance
Substitute Rice salad; tomato salad; 2 glasses wine; fresh orange juice

Afternoon tea

Normal Ginger biscuit; tea

Stop Ginger biscuit

Substitute *Ryvita and flavoured cottage cheese; tea

Dinner

Normal 3 measures spirit; Chinese take-away; 2 glasses wine; coffee; mint

Stop Junk food Chinese dishes, coffee in excess of allowance

Substitute 3 measures spirit (if you must); fish and chips; 2 glasses wine; *hot spiced orange juice

SATURDAY

Breakfast

Normal Sausage sandwich; coffee

Stop Sausage sandwich

Substitute Orange segmented and garnished with roasted almonds; coffee; sparkling mineral water

Elevenses

Normal Doughnut; coffee

Stop Doughnut

Substitute Banana; coffee

Lunch

Normal Pub lunch of white bread, cheese, chutney, salad, chips; ½ pint shandy

Stop White bread, chutney

Substitute Pub lunch of granary rolls, butter, cheese, salad, fresh tomatoes, chips; ½ pint shandy

Afternoon tea

Normal Cake; tea

Stop Cake

Substitute Honey and cottage cheese sandwiches made with soda bread; tea

Dinner

Normal 2 measures spirit; avocado filled with prawns; steak; peas; baked potato; grilled tomatoes and mushrooms; ice-cream; 3 glasses wine

Stop Ice-cream

Substitute 2 measures spirit (it is Saturday, after all); avocado filled with prawns; steak; peas; baked potato; grilled tomatoes and mushrooms; fresh fruit salad; wine; sparkling mineral water

SUNDAY

Breakfast

Normal Factory-farmed bacon; sausage; fried bread; grilled tomatoes; orange juice; coffee

Stop Factory-farmed bacon, sausage

Substitute Open-farmed bacon; scrambled eggs; fried bread; grilled tomatoes; fresh squeezed orange juice; coffee

No elevenses today

Lunch

Normal 2 measures spirit; pre-packed roast pork; mashed potato; cabbage; peas; gravy; home-made apple pie with cream; coffee

Stop Pre-packed pork

Substitute 2 measures spirit; organic pork; mashed potato; cabbage; peas; gravy; home-made apple pie with cream; coffee

Afternoon tea

Normal Biscuit; tea

Stop Biscuit

Substitute 1 slice toasted soda bread with honey; tea

Dinner

Normal Spanish omelette; salad; bread; cheese; celery; 2 glasses wine
Stop Food None
Substitute None

WHAT NEXT?

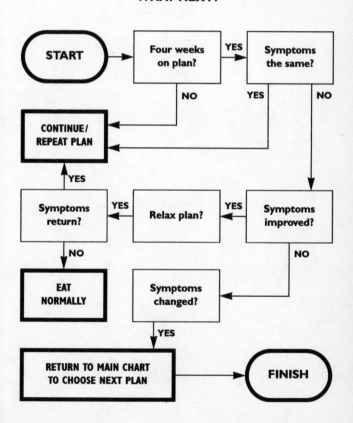

6. The Menstrual Syndrome Eating Plan

MENSTRUAL SYNDROME PLAN CHECK CHART

Before you start the Menstrual Syndrome Eating Plan, fill in the check chart below by ticking any Yes answers to double-check you have chosen the most appropriate plan.

1. I am female. ☐
2. My symptoms are markedly worse in the 10 days or so leading up to my period. ☐
3. My husband, family and close friends can tell when my period is due. ☐
4. My weight increases before my period and decreases afterwards. ☐
5. I am often over-emotional (e.g. cry easily) for no apparent reason. ☐
6. I feel bloated most of the time. ☐
7. I am prone to migraines around the time of my period. ☐
8. I can eat my way through a box of chocolates. ☐
9. I drink a lot of coffee. ☐
10. My periods are heavy and/or generally problematic. ☐

Ticks KEY

0–3 You are in danger of misinterpreting more general dietary problems as being due to menstrual syndrome. The temptation is to look out for symptoms only at certain times of the month and ignore them at other times if they don't fit in. Overcome this by keeping a daily diary of how you feel for a couple of months, then look back and see if your symptoms really do coincide with your menstrual cycle. While you are keeping your diary go on the Low-processing Eating Plan (p. 152), which will keep you generally healthy.

4–8 The Menstrual Syndrome Eating Plan may well help you. If you answered Yes to 10, ask for a Well-Woman check from your family doctor as you may have a medical problem.

9–10 Again, you are in danger of assuming your problems are period-associated when they may not be. For example, if you answered Yes to 6, it is more likely that your bloating is due to candida than to pre-menstrual fluid retention, so have a look at the Anti-candida Eating Plan (p. 228). If you answered Yes to 8, it is likely that your most pressing need is the Low-sugar Eating Plan.

WELCOME TO THE MENSTRUAL SYNDROME EATING PLAN

Since you have chosen this eating plan, you are obviously a menstrual syndrome sufferer and you don't need me to tell you just how debilitating and unpleasant the condition can be. However, while women have lived with menstrual syndrome for centuries, it has only been in the last 30 years or so that it has been medically recognised and explored. Even now there is a great deal of ignorance and confusion surrounding menstrual syndrome. So it makes sense to start the Menstrual Syndrome Eating Plan by taking a close look at the current thinking on the condition and clarifying some of the differing views taken of it.

The first difficulty has been in giving menstrual syndrome an accurate name. It has been referred to by women for years as 'The Curse', 'period pains', 'monthlies', etc. Even in Elizabethan times the Queen was known to be indisposed at certain times – historians think she often used this as a political weapon when she wanted to retreat from difficult diplomatic situations.

More recently, doctors have given the name dysmenorrhoea to the most commonly known and easily diagnosed menstruation problem, that of abdominal cramps and flu-like symptoms lasting two or three days from the onset of menstruation. Nearly every woman has suffered dysmenorrhoea at some time in her life. Unfortunately it very often happens in the mid to late-teens – just the time when girls are taking exams and laying the foundations of their career.

There has never really been any problem in gaining medical acceptance for this manifestation of menstrual syndrome. It is now frequently treated with oral contraceptives to replace cyclical menstruation with 'pseudo-menstruation', which is far less prone to reproduce the symptoms of dysmenorrhoea.

Other forms of menstrual syndrome, however, are equally common. As women get older, they very often begin to notice a vaguer, less dramatic, but equally upsetting range of symptoms: moodiness, tearfulness, irritability, headaches, tiredness, depression, swollen hips and abdomen, tender breasts – pre-period blues, in other words.

It has always been known that these symptoms occur and are linked with menstruation – this is one of the reasons why so many cultures regard women as physically and morally inferior to men. But from a medical point of view it has always been extremely difficult to make a clinical description of such a diffuse syndrome. It has been equally hard to pinpoint it through experiment, since the symptoms and their cycle vary so widely that it is almost impossible to establish scientific controls.

Two major changes in circumstances in the second half of this century changed the situation. First of all the arrival of oral contraception meant that large numbers of young women began to control their menstrual cycles: either arresting them completely, going through 'pseudo-menstruation', or going through phases of ovulating and not ovulating. The artificial 28-day cycle of oral contraception also made women more accurately aware of their bodily cycles. This meant that more detailed observation of cyclical symptoms and their connection with natural menstruation was possible.

The second milestone has been the sustained and brilliant work of the gynaecologist Dr Katharina Dalton. Her clinical definitions of menstrual syndrome have now been so widely accepted that they have been used as a defence in court cases. With the publicity surrounding these court cases in the 1980s some confusion arose over what menstrual syndrome actually was. The term PMT, pre-menstrual tension, was used. This emphasised the emotional 'tension' aspects of menstrual syndrome rather than the wider biological condition. This almost certainly did women a disservice, since the mass media view tended to be: 'Women go mad before their periods and that's a medical fact.'

In an effort to counter this one-sided attitude and to stress the physiological aspects of the syndrome (and of course its physical treatment), gynaecologists and women's organisations now encourage the use of the phrase PMS, pre-menstrual syndrome. This emphasises the fact that the condition has a wide syndrome of symptoms which may or may not appear in the form of emotional trauma.

However, I believe there is now also a case for dropping 'pre-' from the title. 'Pre-' suggests that menstrual syndrome only occurs in the week just before the onset of menstruation. But current research now points to there being symptoms that occur around ovulation, between ovulation and menstruation, during menstruation, and even, rarely, in the days after menstruation (though these may be an after-effect of physical trauma suffered during menstruation). Therefore it is more accurate simply to refer to 'menstrual syndrome' – in other words a variety of symptoms whose occurrence is observed to be linked to the female menstrual cycle.

The table below shows the three main occurrences of menstrual syndrome:

Forms of Menstrual Syndrome

Acute　　　　　The earliest form to be recognised by doctors.
Commonly known as 'period pains' (medical name:
spasmodic dysmenorrhoea). Backache, sickness and
abdominal cramps with onset on the morning of
menstruation. Clears up by about day 3.

Generalised　　A profuse and changing range of symptoms with onset
at any time in the cycle, though usually worse just
before and during menstruation. Hard to diagnose.

PMS　　　　　　Pre-menstrual syndrome. Currently the most
investigated form. A range of grouped symptoms with
onset from ovulation onwards but not evident in the
week after menstruation.

In addition to the three main forms of menstrual syndrome there
are also four groups of symptoms which researchers have now
recognised as having distinct separate causes. Many sufferers
display just one of the symptom groups, while others have
evidence of a couple of symptom groups. It is fortunately rare for
all four groups to be suffered at the same time.

Here is a table of the four main symptom groups, showing the
biological sources of the symptoms and the role diet plays in
producing them.

Four Menstrual Syndrome Symptom Groups

Group	Symptoms	Biological Link	Food Problem
Group A	Headache, temper, dizziness, poor concentration, anxiety, cravings	Blood sugar levels	Sugar, high sugar products

Group B	Bloatedness, tender breasts, backache	Fluid retention	Salt, highly processed foods, high carbohydrate, insufficient water consumption
Group C	Tiredness, weakness, depression	Trace element imbalance	Highly processed foods, diuretics, alcohol, caffeine
Group D	Asthma, cold sores, migraine	Low immune levels	Highly processed foods, artificial food additives, insufficient fresh fruit and vegetables

If you suspect you are a menstrual syndrome sufferer, the first thing to do is get as accurate a picture as possible of just what form your menstrual syndrome takes.

There are two questions you need to ask yourself:

- Which form of menstrual syndrome do I suffer?
- What symptom group or groups do I experience?

To be accurate about this you will need to keep a symptom diary. Get hold of one of those calendars that has a month at a view, with blank squares for you to fill in appointments. Use it to keep a daily record of your symptoms.

To make it easier to see the pattern of your symptoms, use a different coloured crayon or felt tip for each different symptom. You will need to keep this chart for at least three months, but if you feel like commencing the Menstrual Syndrome Eating Plan right from the start, you can. If it immediately alleviates your symptoms you will be able to record this in the symptom diary, but if not you will be able to get a more accurate picture of exactly which elements of the eating plan are most relevant to you. Keep your symptom diary going whether you are on or off the eating plan (but make clear in the diary which is which).

The Menstrual Syndrome Eating Plan is a general nutritional approach designed to combat all the different symptom groups associated with the syndrome. In following the plan you need to be extremely methodical in monitoring both your food intake and your symptoms. The syndrome can fluctuate so much that even clinicians find it hard to monitor, so you will need to be as scientific as you can. Now read on to find out how the Menstrual Syndrome Eating Plan works.

HOW IT WORKS

The Menstrual Syndrome Eating Plan is going to be about the healthiest eating of your life. Since research has shown sufferers to be sensitive to sugars, highly refined and processed foods, caffeine, and poor nutrition, this eating plan contains lots of imaginative but nutritious substitutes for these foods.

Emotional problems are a major factor in menstrual syndrome, so it is very important that any diet you follow doesn't contribute to depression and mood swings by making you feel hungry and deprived. Therefore the Menstrual Syndrome Eating Plan doesn't count calories or measure foods at all. Nor does it prohibit you from eating. Instead you can eat as much as you want, and lots of tasty and treat foods are included. There's no ban on eating out or take-away either, since this can be exactly the time when you need those most.

The simple rule of the eating plan is to remove from your eating those foods which will contribute to your symptoms and replace them with equally satisfying, nourishing and tasty foods which will not pose any problems for you. The eating plan is amazingly simple to follow. Just read through the Step-by-step Guide (p. 190) and you're off!

EXTRA HELP FOR MENSTRUAL SYNDROME

Most researchers now feel diet is the major contributor to menstrual syndrome symptoms, and the work of the Women's Nutritional Advisory Service (for address see p. 337) has helped thousands of women feel better by adjusting their eating. However, because of the emotional factors inherent in menstrual syndrome it's a good idea to make some lifestyle changes as well.

Exercise

Some excellent research has shown that regular medium level exercise is very helpful, particularly against acute and generalised forms of menstrual syndrome. A brisk hour's outdoor walk every other day is excellent, as is regular swimming. Joining an exercise class is a good idea as well, because its social element can improve mood and distract from symptoms.

Family

Explain about menstrual syndrome as clearly as you can to your husband and family. If it helps, show them this chapter so they can read about it for themselves. If everybody knows what is going on it is much easier to keep it in its place and prevent it from spoiling other areas of your life.

Relaxation

Those who suffer particularly from Group A and Group C symptoms (see pp. 185 and 186) find relaxation techniques very helpful. You can get details of local yoga and relaxation classes from your council information office or the local paper or newsagent.

In more severe cases counselling and therapy can also help – it may be that your emotional menstrual syndrome is linked to some other trauma in your life of which you may not be fully aware. You can get details of counselling from your family doctor, or look at the addresses on pp. 336 and 337.

Breathing

One easily learnt technique for improving well-being is the 'breathe and see' method. It need only take a couple of minutes as often as you feel you need it. Here's a step-by-step approach to it:

1 Find a quiet place where you can be alone for a minute or so (the loo is where I usually take refuge!).
2 Sit comfortably and loosen your waistband if it is tight.
3 Close your eyes.
4 Place your hand on your diaphragm (the wide hollow just above your navel where your ribs separate and tail off).
5 Slowly take air into your body, feeling your diaphragm lift and push against your hand as you do so.
6 Hold it for a second.
7 Gently use your hand to press down on your diaphragm and slowly squeeze the air out of your body.
8 Now try again without using your hand. You should feel your diaphragm working properly (perhaps for the first time!). In future you won't need your hand to help you breathe correctly, but at first it gives you a good idea how it should feel.
9 Do this once or twice a day for a few days until you are used to it.
10 Now you can add the 'see' element. While you are breathing, with your eyes closed, visualise yourself in the most pleasant place you can imagine. It might be on a silver sand beach in the West Indies; or it might be on the Yorkshire Moors on a bright blustery morning; anywhere, indoors or outdoors – choose what you want.
11 As you breathe, sense what it is like to be in this ideal place. Get a detailed picture of the view. What is the

weather? Is it warm? What does it smell and sound like?
Use every sense to appreciate this beautiful place.

12 Now tune in to how you feel here in this lovely spot. You
are comfortable, relaxed and happy. It is the ideal place to
be. There is nothing worrying you, you feel utterly calm.

13 As you begin to feel rested and relaxed you can feel your
energy and optimism flooding back. You know that when
you eventually leave you will feel well and capable of
coping with life.

14 When you are ready to complete the exercise (usually after
a couple of minutes) open your eyes. Stand up and stretch.
Off you go.

STEP-BY-STEP GUIDE TO THE MENSTRUAL SYNDROME EATING PLAN

1   Read all sections of the diet carefully.

2   Learn what the stop foods are and why you must stop them.

3   Get familiar with all the substitutes and where to buy them.

4   Go through the week-long sample eating programme and work out
how it will fit into your lifestyle.

5   If you are at all uncertain you can decide to follow the sample eating
programme exactly for a week until you get the hang of things.

6   Learn how to make the snack substitutes.

7   Make a copy of the glance guide to stop and substitute foods.

8   Take the glance guide shopping with you to make sure you are
stocking up on the right foods.

9   Remember that any food not mentioned as a stop food can be eaten
whenever you like.

10 Note which drinks are to be stopped.

11 Eat plenty of fresh vegetables – these are not stop foods.

12 Follow the diet for at least 2 months before reviewing your
symptoms and deciding whether to continue on it, change to another
diet, or return to normal eating.

STOP, THINK, SUBSTITUTE

Which foods should I stop eating and what should I substitute?

Complex Carbohydrate Group

Carbohydrate metabolism plays an important part in menstrual
syndrome. A diet too high in refined carbohydrate (sugar)
contributes to the swings in blood sugar level which are a
prominent feature in menstrual syndrome. But the consumption
of complex carbohydrates helps to even out blood sugar levels
because complex carbohydrates are metabolised more slowly
than refined carbohydrates.

So the menstrual syndrome eating planner should aim to
browse frequently on complex carbohydrates, both at regular
mealtimes and as between meal snacks.

The best sources of complex carbohydrate are whole grains
(wheat, oats, rye, etc.); rice; potatoes and root vegetables; beans
and pulses. Ordinary wheat bread, though, is not recommended
at first for menstrual syndrome eating planners because it is more
quickly digested by the body into simple sugars. Also some
menstrual syndrome sufferers have a tendency towards allergy
which may be triggered by wheat. For these reasons, cut out
wheat breads and pastas to begin with and then reintroduce
them when your symptoms are stable enough for you to see if
you are affected by wheat.

- **Stop:** Wheat bread; pasta.

- **Substitute:** Continental rye and sourdough breads; rice.

Refined Carbohydrate Group

It is very important for menstrual syndrome sufferers to replace the refined carbohydrates in their diet by substituting an increased intake of both complex carbohydrates and protein. This will have the important effect of stabilising erratic blood sugar levels. Refined carbohydrate is the nutritional name for sugar. Excessive intake of sugar contributes to the hypoglycaemic syndrome that we discussed earlier, so it is very important to substitute not just sugar in your diet but all sugar containing foods.

Many manufactured sugar foods like cakes and biscuits often also include sodium bicarbonate, which is a salt form, and therefore should be avoided because of the threat it poses to maintaining fluid balances.

- **Stop**: Sugar, syrups; confectionery; cakes; biscuits; commercial puddings and desserts.

- **Substitute**: Sparing honey and fresh fruit juice for spreading and sweetening; fresh fruit; continental bread spread with diet fromage frais; rice cakes spread with cottage cheese; home-made fruit pies.

Protein Group

A regular, adequate intake of protein is very important, since the digestion of protein provides amino acids which contribute to balanced hormonal function. Among the complex of factors involved in menstrual syndrome, hormonal malfunction is one of the most prominent.

Protein is available from meat, fish, beans and pulses, rice, soya bean, eggs, nuts and cheese. However, some of these protein sources also include salts – sodium, sodium nitrate, monosodium glutamate and sodium bicarbonate (especially in convenience foods) – so some protein sources must be substituted.

Meaty junk foods contain salts, sugar and fats, which negates their protein value for the menstrual syndrome planner.

- **Stop:** Salted nuts; bacon; salted fish and meats (including kippers); junk food; Chinese take-away; ham; tinned meat soups.

- **Substitute:** Raw vegetable sticks; thin cut grilled pork; plain fish and meats; sandwiches; Greek take-away; cold chicken; home-made soup.

Vegetable and Fruit Group

Most of the foods in this group are very helpful to menstrual syndrome. They are often rich sources of the vitamins, minerals and trace elements which are vital in combating symptoms. Nor in their natural state do they contain the refined sugars, salts and saturated fats that cause difficulties for menstrual syndrome sufferers.

But fruits are a source of simple sugars (natural refined carbohydrate) and this provokes a difference of opinion in nutritionists. Some are quite happy for fruits to be eaten ad lib since the sugar they contain is present along with a large amount of water and fibre. Others believe that as a source of sugar their intake should be limited.

I take the middle line. I think you can eat plenty of the less sugary fruits (the less sweet ones). Experiment with the watery sugary fruits (such as melon) to see what effect they have on you personally. Cut out completely dried fruits and those adulterated during processing. Bananas are problematic because they have high potassium levels which are helpful to the menstrual syndrome planner, but they are also a source of amines, excess of which can be a problem for some menstrual syndrome sufferers. Personally, I find bananas very useful, but your body may react differently.

- **Stop**: Potato crisps; tinned vegetables; deep-fried
  vegetables; chips; tinned vegetable soups; canned and dried
  fruits; salted olives.

- **Substitute**: Raw vegetable sticks; fresh/frozen vegetables;
  steamed/raw/stir-fried vegetables; jacket potatoes; home-
  made soup; fresh fruit; unsalted olives. *Note*: chips fried in
  sunflower oil can be eaten.

Dairy Group

The dairy group creates two main problems. One is its saturated
fat content, which may play a role in disrupting the prostaglandin cycle. More apparent is the fact that dairy products are so
often presented in products which also contain high quantities of
sugar and salt. Chocolate is an obvious example, where not just
sugar but caffeine too pose problems for the menstrual syndrome
sufferer. Other dairy products such as cheese often contain salt
(sometimes sodium nitrate too) which causes fluid retention.

- **Stop**: Chocolates; malted drinks; ice-cream; smoked cheese;
  hard cheese.

- **Substitute**: Sandwiches (especially crispbread sandwiches);
  warm soya milk with vanilla essence; frozen yoghurt;
  cottage cheese; Edam/Gouda cheese.

Fats Group and EFAs

Essential fatty acids are the building blocks from which the body
generates prostaglandins. Most doctors and nutritionists now
believe that lack of prostaglandins, and imbalance of the
prostaglandin cycle, is implicated in most cases of menstrual
syndrome.

The best sources of EFAs are plant oils, especially sunflower
oil and safflower oil (and evening primrose oil, which is too
expensive to cook with). But not only do most fats not supply

EFAs, many saturated fats are even believed to disrupt the process by which EFAs are converted into prostaglandins.

Another problem is that although most vegetable margarines claim to be high in polyunsaturated fats (the group which includes EFA yielding oils), the chemical process which alters these fats (to make them solid at room temperature) decreases the amount of EFA available from the product. So it is a good idea to switch to fresh nut, vegetable and seed oils (you can even pick up the Mediterranean habit of dipping bread in oil rather than buttering it).

Some research studies have implicated a high intake of saturated animal fat in the breast tenderness symptom of menstrual syndrome, and one recent study even went so far as to suggest that this may be a factor in breast cancer.

- **Stop:** Vegetable margarines (unless marked high in linoleic acid); lard/dripping.

- **Substitute:** Vegetable oils high in linoleic and gamma-linoleic acids, including sunflower and starflower oil.

Condiments

The bloating and fluid retention symptoms that are so uncomfortable in menstrual syndrome are linked with high salt intake and a low fibre diet. The most obvious source of high concentration of salts (usually accompanied by no fibre) is the condiment group, which should be avoided. There are plenty of natural condiment alternatives which are equally tasty.

- **Stop:** Jam; salt; tomato ketchup; relishes; commercial stock cubes, sauces and gravy mixes; commercial dips.

- **Substitute:** Sparing honey; sesame oil/home-made stock; 'low-salt'/herbs; tomato purée; home-made vegetable purées; pan reduction sauces; home-made yoghurt/avocado dip.

Beverages

Most nutritionists believe that the adrenalin response (which raises blood sugar levels rapidly and temporarily) is a major factor in menstrual syndrome. The hypoglycaemic syndrome (where blood sugar falls abnormally low) is one trigger of the adrenalin response. Increasingly, though, doctors believe that the adrenalin response can be triggered by other factors. Stress is one of them. Other dietary triggers include alcohol, caffeine and possibly theobromine. It therefore makes sense to avoid sources of these substances.

- **Stop**: Alcohol; tea; coffee; chocolate drinks; fizzy drinks; colas; sweetened fruit juices.

- **Substitute**: Mineral water; diet tonic water; herbal/fruit teas; hot bouillon; diet bitter lemon; diet ginger beer; tomato juice/fresh-squeezed juices.

Eating Out and Take-away

Psychologically, eating out is probably a very good idea for the menstrual syndrome sufferer. It alleviates the stress of having to prepare a meal; if enjoyed with family and friends it promotes a sense of companionship and involvement; it can be very relaxing.

But when you are eating out, remember your eating plan and stick to it as closely as possible. Choose simple dishes, and, if you can afford it, go to a restaurant where you know the food will be fresh and well-cooked. Avoid alcohol, sugar, high fat and salt.

Take-aways usually contain such a high junk food element that they are not advisable for the menstrual syndrome planner. Chinese take-away often has a lot of salt, sugar and monosodium glutamate in it. Indian take-away may be high in fat. Of all the take-aways good old fish and chips will probably be best tolerated (as long as you don't have the chips too salty), and well-cooked Greek take-away is generally the healthiest.

AT-A-GLANCE GUIDE TO STOP AND SUBSTITUTE FOODS

Stop – *Substitute*

Complex Carbohydrate Food Group

bread – *continental rye and sourdough breads*
pasta – *rice*

Refined Carbohydrate Food Group

sugar – *limited honey*
syrups – *fresh fruit juice*
confectionery – *fresh fruit*
cakes – *continental bread spread with diet fromage frais*
biscuits – *rice cakes spread with cottage cheese*
commercial puddings and desserts – *home-made fruit pies*

Protein Food Group

salted nuts – *raw vegetable sticks*

bacon – *thin cut grilled pork*
salted fish and meats – *plain fish and meat*
kippers – *fresh fish/tuna in olive oil*
junk food – *sandwiches*
Chinese take-away – *Greek take-away*
ham – *cold chicken*
tinned meat soups – *home-made soup*

Vegetable and Fruit Food Group

potato crisps – *unsalted olives/raw vegetable sticks*
tinned vegetables – *fresh/frozen vegetables*
fried vegetables – *steamed/raw vegetables*
chips – *jacket potatoes*
tinned vegetable soups – *home-made soup*
canned fruits – *fresh fruit*
salted olives – *unsalted olives*

Dairy Food Group

full fat milk – *soya milk*

chocolates – see Snack Substitutes (p. 313)

malted drinks – *warm soya milk with vanilla essence*

ice-cream – *frozen yoghurt*

smoked cheese – *plain cottage cheese*

hard cheese – *Edam/Gouda cheese*

tomato ketchup – *tomato purée*

relishes – *home-made vegetable purées*

commercial stock cubes – *home-made stock*

commercial sauce and gravy mix – *pan reduction sauces*

commercial dips – *home-made yoghurt/avocado dip*

Fats Group

vegetable margarine – *olive oil*

dripping/lard – *sunflower oil/safflower oil*

Condiments

jam – *trace honey/fruit purée*

salt – *'low-salt'/herbs*

Beverages

alcohol – *mineral water/Piermont/diet tonic water*

tea – *herbal/fruit teas*

coffee – *hot bouillon*

fizzy drinks – *mineral water*

colas – *diet bitter lemon/diet ginger beer*

sweetened fruit juices – *tomato juice/ fresh-squeeze juices*

SAMPLE SUBSTITUTION PROGRAMME

* Items marked with an asterisk are given in greater detail in the Snack Substitutes and Recipes sections (pp. 313, 324).

MONDAY

Breakfast

Normal 2 slices wholemeal toast with butter and marmalade; cereal with milk; sweetened orange juice; coffee with milk and sugar

Includes these Stop Foods Wholemeal bread, sweetened orange juice, coffee, sugar

Substitute 2 slices rye bread toast with butter and honey; cereal (preferably without sugar, check pack) with milk; fresh squeezed orange juice; *hot lemon juice with honey

Elevenses

Normal 1 biscuit; coffee with milk and sugar

Stop Biscuit, coffee, sugar

Substitute *1 plain oatcake; *hot bouillon

Lunch

Normal Bowl of soup; sausage roll and salad; apple; 1 glass wine

Stop Sausage roll, wine

Substitute Bowl of soup; tuna and salad; apple; sparkling mineral water

Afternoon tea

Normal Piece of cake; cup of tea without sugar

Stop Cake, tea

Substitute *2 rice cakes spread with flavoured diet fromage frais; *hot spiced orange juice

Dinner

Normal Prawn cocktail with 2 slices brown bread; pasta in tomato sauce with courgettes; ice-cream

Stop Brown bread, pasta, ice-cream

Substitute Prawn cocktail with 2 Ryvitas; *risotto with tomatoes and herbs; courgettes; *plain yoghurt mashed with frozen raspberries

TUESDAY

Breakfast

Normal 1 soft-boiled egg with 2 slices white bread and butter; fresh orange juice; coffee

Stop White bread, coffee

Substitute 1 soft-boiled egg with 2 Ryvitas and butter; fresh orange juice; *hot lemon juice and honey

Elevenses

Normal American-style cookie; coffee

Stop Cookie, coffee

Substitute Orange; *hot skimmed milk with vanilla essence

Lunch

Normal Fried chicken limb in breadcrumbs; chips; peas; individual portion fruit trifle; 1 glass wine; coffee

Stop Breadcrumbs, trifle, wine, coffee

Substitute Plain chicken limb (or scrape off breadcrumbs); chips; peas; fruit salad with yoghurt; sparkling mineral water

Afternoon tea

Normal Small bar of chocolate; tea

Stop Chocolate, tea

Substitute *Banana and Ryvita sandwich; *hot bouillon

Dinner

Normal Packet of potato crisps; sausages; baked beans; 2 slices white toast; flavoured jelly; 2 glasses wine; coffee; 1 chocolate truffle

Stop Potato crisps, sausages, baked beans, toast, jelly, wine, truffle, coffee

Substitute Handful of olives or raw vegetable sticks; grilled continental sausage; *home-cooked mixed pulses in fresh tomato sauce; 2 slices oven-warmed continental bread; portion plain creamy yoghurt sprinkled with honey and walnuts; *Piermont; *hot lemon juice with honey; tangerine

WEDNESDAY

Breakfast

Normal Cereal with milk; pancake with maple syrup; fresh squeezed orange juice; coffee

Stop Maple syrup, coffee

Substitute Cereal with milk; pancake with butter and honey; fresh squeezed orange juice; *hot skimmed milk with vanilla essence

Elevenses

Normal Shortcake biscuit; coffee

Stop Shortcake biscuit, coffee

Substitute *Rice cake spread with flavoured cottage cheese; *hot spiced orange juice

Lunch

Normal Scotch egg salad; 2 slices brown bread; apple; wine; coffee

Stop Scotch egg, brown bread, wine, coffee

Substitute 2 slices cold beef; large continental salad; 2 slices crispbread; orange; mineral water

Afternoon tea

Normal Snack bar; tea

Stop Snack bar, tea

Substitute *Oatcake; *hot bouillon

Dinner

Normal Bowl of soup; grilled lamb chop; spinach; mashed potato; tomato purée; fresh unsugared fruit salad; hot lemon juice with honey

Stop None

Substitute None

THURSDAY

Breakfast

Normal 2 rashers of bacon and 1 fried egg on white toast; fresh orange juice; coffee

Stop Bacon, toast, coffee

Substitute Fried onions and mushrooms; 1 fried egg on a thick slice of continental bread; fresh orange juice; *hot lemon juice and honey

Elevenses

Normal Chocolate digestive biscuit; coffee

Stop Biscuit, coffee

Substitute *2 Ryvitas spread with honey and flavoured cottage cheese; *hot spiced orange juice

Lunch

Normal Baked potato with cheese; salad; chocolate gâteau; coffee; Coca Cola

Stop Chocolate gâteau, coffee, Coca Cola

Substitute Baked potato with cheese; salad; *mashed banana with yoghurt and crumbled oatcake; mineral water; *hot bouillon

Afternoon tea

Normal Egg sandwich; tea

Stop White bread, tea

Substitute 2 slices Ryvita sandwiched round sliced egg and tomato; *hot bouillon

Dinner

Normal Taramasalata with brown bread; commercially prepared cod and salmon fish pie; spinach; grilled tomatoes; ice-cream; 2 glasses wine; coffee; after-dinner mint

Stop Brown bread, ice-cream, wine, coffee

Substitute Taramasalata with water biscuits; if fish pie contains sugar, then *home-made fish pie, otherwise don't worry; *frozen yoghurt; *Piermont; kiwi fruit

FRIDAY

Breakfast

Normal Toast with jam; coffee

Stop Toast, jam, coffee

Substitute 2 rice cakes spread with butter and honey; fresh orange juice; *hot lemon juice with honey

Elevenses

Normal Apple, coffee

Stop Coffee

Substitute Apple; *hot bouillon

Lunch

Normal Pork pie with chutney; tomato salad; 2 glasses wine; coffee

Stop Pork pie, chutney, wine, coffee

Substitute Rice salad; tomato salad; fresh orange juice; sparkling mineral water

Afternoon tea

Normal Ginger biscuit; tea

Stop Ginger biscuit, tea

Substitute *Ryvita and flavoured cottage cheese; *hot bouillon

Dinner

Normal 3 measures spirit; Chinese take-away; 2 glasses wine; coffee; mint

Stop Spirits, Chinese take-away, wine, coffee

Substitute *2 Virgin Marys; Greek take-away; sparkling mineral water; orange quarters

SATURDAY

Breakfast

Normal I slice toast; coffee

Stop Toast, coffee

Substitute Orange segmented and garnished with roasted almonds; sparkling mineral water

Elevenses

Normal Doughnut; coffee

Stop Doughnut, coffee

Substitute Egg custard tart; fresh orange juice. While not ideal, the egg custard is a good compromise for the weekend.

Lunch

Normal Pub lunch of bread, cheese, chutney, salad, chips; ½ pint shandy

Stop Bread, chutney, chips, shandy

Substitute Pub lunch of gammon with pineapple; salad; baked potato; tomato juice

Afternoon tea

Normal Cake; tea

Stop Cake, tea

Substitute Honey and cottage cheese sandwiches made with rye bread; *hot spiced orange juice

Dinner

Normal 2 measures spirit; avocado filled with prawns; steak; peas; baked potato; grilled tomatoes and mushrooms; ice-cream; 3 glasses wine

Stop Spirits, ice-cream, wine

Substitute *2 Virgin Marys; avocado filled with prawns; steak; peas; baked potato; grilled tomatoes and mushrooms; fresh fruit salad; sparkling mineral water

SUNDAY

Breakfast

Normal Bacon; sausage; fried white bread; grilled tomatoes; orange juice; coffee

Stop Bacon, sausage, bread, coffee

Substitute Large open mushrooms stuffed with butter and parsley and grilled; grilled continental sausage slices; toasted rye bread; grilled tomatoes; fresh squeezed orange juice; *hot lemon juice with honey

No elevenses today

Lunch

Normal 2 measures spirit; roast pork; mashed potato; cabbage; peas; gravy mix gravy; apple pie with cream; coffee

Stop Spirits, gravy mix, coffee

Substitute *2 Virgin Marys; roast pork; mashed potato; cabbage; peas; pan juice gravy; apple pie with cream; *hot spiced orange juice

Afternoon tea

Normal Biscuit; tea

Stop Biscuit, tea

Substitute 1 slice toasted rye bread with honey; *hot lemon juice with honey

Dinner

Normal Spanish omelette; salad; bread; cheese; celery; 2 glasses wine

Stop Bread, wine

Substitute Spanish omelette; salad; oven-warmed rye bread; cheese; celery; *Piermont

WHAT NEXT?

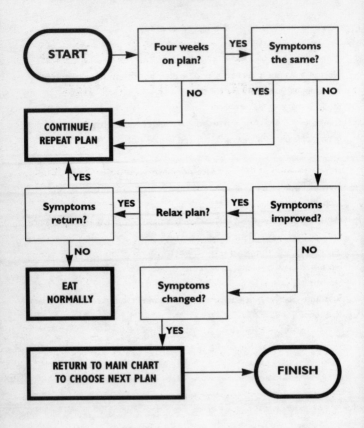

7. The Oral Contraceptive Syndrome Eating Plan

ORAL CONTRACEPTIVE SYNDROME PLAN CHECK CHART

Before you start the Oral Contraceptive Syndrome Eating Plan, fill in the check chart below by ticking any Yes answers to double-check that you have chosen the most appropriate eating plan.

1. I have been taking oral contraceptives more than 6 months. ☐
2. I feel constantly tired and run-down. ☐
3. Friends have commented that I seem depressed. ☐
4. I am always on a diet or starting a new one. ☐
5. I am fatter than I ought to be. ☐
6. My breasts feel tender. ☐
7. My skin is red and flaky especially round nose and mouth. ☐
8. I eat a lot of junk food. ☐
9. I get a lot of headaches. ☐
10. I've become prone to thrush. ☐

Ticks KEY

0–3 The vast majority of women taking oral contraceptives find their health is unaffected. Provided you have regular Well Woman checks it is extremely unlikely that oral contraceptives are contributing to your problems. Go back to the flow chart and think more carefully about your answers.

4–8   For some women oral contraceptives do have general health
          drawbacks. If serious, they can be cured by changing the oral
          contraceptive prescribed. If mild, the Oral Contraceptive Eating Plan
          can be very effective in dealing with symptoms and raising general
          health levels.

9–10 Be careful not to put pre-existing unsatisfactory health down to the
          fact that you have started taking the Pill. If you answered Yes to 4 or
          8, it is likely that your nutritional state is poor anyway, so try the
          Low-processing Eating Plan (p. 152) first.

IMPORTANT: Some medical conditions make oral contraception
an unsuitable method for certain women. When you approach
your family planning doctor for a prescription, make sure he or
she knows everything about you and your family's medical
background. For an excellent detailed source of information
about taking oral contraception, read *The Pill Protection Plan*
(details in bibliography, p. 341).

WELCOME TO THE ORAL CONTRACEPTIVE
SYNDROME EATING PLAN

A whole generation of women has now grown up taking the Pill
and yet still the debate rumbles on about whether or not oral
contraception is a good idea. If like me you're in your 30s, you've
probably been on and off various different Pill brands more often
than you can remember. You've just settled on a brand that
doesn't leave you looking like a barrage balloon, when along
comes another scare story and it's back to struggling with the live
goldfish syndrome (you know, the one where the diaphragm
leaps across the bathroom like a salmon going up a waterfall).

To the unbiased observer there are actually very few serious
medical risks associated with oral contraception – far fewer, in

fact, than there are to giving birth. But the trouble is that the Pill has become politicised over the years. At first feminists were great supporters of oral contraception because it enabled women to enjoy sexual activity without risk of becoming responsible for the upbringing of a child. Nowadays the issue is less straightforward. The connection of oral contraception with increased risk of thrombosis, high blood pressure and possibly some cancers has meant that the Pill is no longer seen as quite the boon it once was. Feminists are now angry that it is women who are expected to take the responsibility for contraception. They think it is unfair that men rarely pay much attention to contraception whereas women are willing to jeopardise their health for it.

Again, this view may soon change once more, since the advent of AIDS has meant that men are becoming more aware of the desirability of responsible sex and are more willing to make the chosen contraceptive method a barrier one.

There is also an extreme viewpoint held by female conspiracy theorists that the Pill was invented by men as a way of gaining ultimate power over women by controlling their menstrual cycles and arresting their fertility. People who believe this sometimes claim that the Pill keeps women immature – that when taking oral contraception their voices are higher, they are less assertive and they display fewer physical and emotional sexual characteristics. There is absolutely no clinical evidence for this whatsoever, but I include it to show just how overstated people can be in their views on oral contraception.

My aim in the Oral Contraceptive Syndrome Eating Plan is to present a picture that is realistic, rational, and above all, helpful to you, the Pill taker. If you have long ago reached the conclusion that the Pill is the most convenient and practical form of contraception for you, then you are to be supported in your decision, not put to needless anxiety through alarmist writing.

So far, reputable clinical research into the Pill has raised various plus and minus attributes as follows:

Decreased Risk	Increased Risk
of ovarian cyst	of uterine fibroid tumour
of ovarian cancer	of breast cancer (under debate)
of endometrial cancer	of thrombosis
	of raised blood pressure

It is important to know that these are 'risk factors', not causes and cures of the diseases mentioned. The risks are not particularly high. Where there is a genuine probability of the Pill contributing to disease, the practitioner will prescribe a different form of contraception. This is particularly stressed in the high blood pressure/thrombosis/sudden migraines area, especially if the patient has a personal or family history of circulation problems.

So, putting aside all the hysteria, there are in fact very few medical reasons why you should not take the Pill.

But that isn't the end of the story. What about the mild, non-medical side effects? What about the weight gain; the breast tenderness; that vague but persistent feeling of being generally under the weather? Since you have chosen this eating plan I am sure you know exactly what I mean.

It's that generalised 'out of sorts' feeling so many Pill takers report, and which I have christened oral contraceptive syndrome. The anecdotal evidence for these mild but often long-lasting side-effects of oral contraception is now so great that it is impossible to ignore.

The first point about oral contraceptive syndrome is that it is not bad enough for you to want to stop taking the Pill. If it is, then you may well have a problem that you should discuss at your next Well Woman clinic. Most people with oral contraceptive syndrome want to go on taking the Pill because they like it as a form of contraception; it would just make life easier if they could feel a little more well.

The good news is that it is very easily possible for you to feel 110 per cent while taking the Pill, and you need make only minor modifications to your eating to achieve this. Excellent research has now been carried out by various dietary supplement companies to discover the biological processes that can cause oral contraceptive syndrome. They have discovered that the effect of the hormones in the Pill is to cause certain minor imbalances in the body's metabolism. The table below shows what causes these imbalances, the symptoms which result and how to correct the imbalance.

Imbalance	Cause	Symptoms	Correction
Zinc availability depleted	Possibly due to Pill raising copper levels	Lowered immune system/colds	Zinc supplement
Higher dietary requirement for B6	Possibly due to raised oestrogen levels stimulating metabolic processes involving B6	Depression/ moodiness (see note on tryptophane cycle)	B complex vitamin supplement
Higher incidence of *candida albicans* overgrowth (thrush)	Possibly due to changed levels of acidity in vagina	Thrush/candidiasis (see Anti-candida Eating Plan, p. 228)	Cut out sugar and yeast
Fluid retention	Prompted by raised oestrogen levels	Breast tenderness/ weight gain	Cut out caffeine/ salt/spicy and fatty foods

NOTE: Tryptophane cycle – Vitamin B6 and tryptophane co-act

in a metabolic process which produces serotonin. Reliable research has shown that serotonin is a major mood influencer, and that low levels are linked with depression. If the body's supplies of B6 are used up by other metabolic functions, not enough remains to trigger the tryptophane cycle. Therefore not enough serotonin is produced and depression may follow.

None of these imbalances is particularly severe, and, as you can see from the table, they can all be remedied by very simple changes in the diet and some supplementation.

The key to the Oral Contraceptive Syndrome Eating Plan is that it is not a restrictive diet. Instead it is more closely related to 'super-nutrition' – the practice of eating for optimum health. Read on to find out how it works.

HOW IT WORKS

Unlike most of the eating plans in this book, there aren't many stop foods. Instead of doing so much stop/substitute you will instead be raising the general quality of your eating. The Oral Contraceptive Syndrome Eating Plan represents a super-healthy diet which is low in the few foods that can trigger imbalances, and high in the foods rich in the extra vitamins and minerals Pill takers need.

Begin by reading the Step-by-step Guide below, and then the rest of the section. Once you've got a good idea of what is involved, you may also find it useful to look at the other high nutrition eating plan in this book, the Special Requirements Eating Plan (p.279), which has a list of the super foods that give you the highest nutritive value with the fewest calories or other adverse dietary elements (fat, sugar, etc.).

These two eating plans – Oral Contraceptive Syndrome and Special Requirements – are perhaps the most exciting in the book because they embody a new concept that is rapidly taking hold of nutritionists, that of 'optimum nutrition'.

Optimum nutrition is the theory that if we eat the healthiest possible diets – high in vitamins, fibre, minerals, trace elements, unsaturated fats and essential fatty acids and at the same time low in saturated fats, sugar, residues, contaminants and additives – our general health and well-being will improve as a result.

So by going on the Oral Contraceptive Syndrome Eating Plan you are blazing a trail towards the nutrition of the twenty-first century. I think I'll join you!

STEP-BY-STEP GUIDE TO THE ORAL CONTRACEPTIVE SYNDROME EATING PLAN

1   Read all sections of the diet carefully.

2   Learn what the stop foods are and why you must stop them.

3   Get familiar with all the substitutes and where to buy them.

4   Go through the week-long sample eating programme and work out how it will fit into your lifestyle.

5   If you are at all uncertain, you can decide to follow the sample eating programme exactly for a week until you get the hang of things.

6   Learn how to make the snack substitutes.

7   Make a copy of the glance guide to stop and substitute foods.

8   Take the glance guide shopping with you to make sure you are stocking up on the right foods.

9   Remember that any food not mentioned as a stop food can be eaten whenever you like.

10   Note which drinks are to be stopped.

11   Eat plenty of fresh vegetables, these are not stop foods.

12   Follow the diet for at least 2 months before reviewing your symptoms and deciding whether to continue on it, change to another diet, or return to normal eating.

STOP, THINK, SUBSTITUTE

Which foods should I stop eating and what should I substitute?

Complex Carbohydrate Group

Complex carbohydrate is basically sugar that comes along with a whole complex of other dietary components – fibre, water, vitamins, minerals, trace elements, some protein – all bound together in a single food product. The complex carbohydrate foods are: cereals (oats, maize, wheat, rye, etc.) and the products made from them (bread, pasta, flour); roots (potatoes, beet, etc.); rice (a cereal crop but unusual in being comparatively high in protein).

Complex carbohydrate is nutritionally different from refined carbohydrate, which is sugar stripped of the rest of its dietary components.

You can easily tell the dietary difference between a complex and a refined carbohydrate product: the complex carbohydrate product will not taste particularly sweet, whereas the refined carbohydrate product will have a sweet taste.

Whereas high consumption of refined carbohydrates contributes to the hypoglycaemia syndrome which can be a problem for those on oral contraception, complex carbohydrate does not. But to begin with you should beware of complex carbohydrates that are very quickly broken down and 'refined' by your body's own digestive system.

A simple experiment to discover this process is to put an ordinary piece of white factory bread in your mouth and chew it for a few moments without swallowing. Almost immediately it begins to taste sweet. That is because your saliva contains an enzyme which rapidly releases the sugar in white bread, long before the digestive process begins in the stomach and gut. Opting for brown bread will slow this down.

- **Stop**: White bread.
- **Substitute**: Brown bread.

Refined Carbohydrate Group

The basic refined carbohydrate is common white sugar. It is refined from complex carbohydrate sources – usually sugar beet or sugar cane. The refining process strips away the complex of other dietary ingredients (fibre, water, vitamins, minerals, etc.) and leaves the simple sugar which is purely a unit of calorific energy without other nutritional ingredients.

A simple sugar can be refined from many different plant-origin complex carbohydrates, but the basic result is always the same: sugar. The different sugars have lots of different names – glucose, sucrose, malt, etc. – but they all amount to much the same thing.

For those on the Oral Contraceptive Syndrome Eating Plan, sugar has two problems. As we have discovered, women on oral contraceptives can sometimes be susceptible to mood swings connected with changes in blood sugar levels. Eating too much sugar makes it extremely difficult to stabilise blood sugar levels, and can aggravate hypoglycaemic conditions.

But for most oral contraceptive syndrome planners, the major problem of sugar is that it is very poor nutritional value for calories, and as we have discovered, the most important element of this plan is high quality nutrition. So get value for calories by cutting down on sugar and substituting foods which are richer in nutrients.

- **Stop**: Sugar, syrup; biscuits; cake; confectionery.
- **Substitute**: Sparing honey/fruit juice for spreading and sweetening; sparing molasses; rice cakes spread with

cottage cheese; continental bread spread with diet fromage frais; fruit.

Protein Group

A regular, adequate intake of protein is important for every balanced diet, but women who suffer from oral contraceptive syndrome seem more prone than others to skimp on their protein intake (nobody is quite sure why). The digestion of protein provides amino acids which contribute to balanced hormonal function.

Protein is available from meat, fish, beans and pulses, rice, soya beans, eggs, nuts and cheese. However, some of these protein sources also include salts – sodium, sodium nitrate, monosodium glutamate and sodium bicarbonate (especially in convenience foods), which may contribute to fluid retention. So it is wise to choose protein sources that are fairly simple and plain.

Meaty junk foods contain not only salts but often sugar as well, which negates their protein value for the oral contraceptive syndrome planner.

- **Stop:** Spiced meats; fried meat and fish; salted nuts; junk food.

- **Substitute:** Plain recipes; grilled/casseroled meat and fish; unsalted nuts; sandwiches.

Vegetable and Fruit Group

Most of the foods in this group are very helpful to the oral contraceptive planner looking for optimum nutrition. They are often rich sources of the vitamins, minerals and trace elements which are vital in combating symptoms. Nor in their natural state do they contain the refined sugars and salts which can cause problems.

- **Stop:** Chips; roast potatoes; tinned vegetables; canned fruit; potato crisps.

- **Substitute:** Stir-fried parsnip and carrot sticks; mashed/ boiled/jacket potatoes; frozen vegetables; fresh fruit; olives/ raw vegetable sticks.

Dairy Group

The oral contraceptive planner shouldn't have too many problems with dairy products, or with fats, except where they have sugar added to make products like chocolate. Obviously the problems that we have noted over sugar then apply.

- **Stop:** Chocolates; malted drinks; chocolate drinks/shakes.

- **Substitute:** Bananas (see Snack Substitutes, p. 313); skimmed milk with vanilla essence; yoghurt and fruit shakes.

Condiments

The bloating and fluid retention symptoms that those taking oral contraceptives can have are linked with high salt intake and low fibre diet. The most obvious source of high concentration of salts (usually accompanied by no fibre) is the condiment group, which should be avoided. There are plenty of natural condiment alternatives which are equally tasty.

- **Stop:** Salt; soy sauce; jam; commercial stock cubes, sauces and gravy mix.

- **Substitute:** 'Low-salt'/herbs; sesame oil/home-made stock; sparing honey; home-made stock and pan reductions.

Beverages

The main aim of the Oral Contraceptive Syndrome Eating Plan is to ensure optimum nutrition generally rather than cut out specific foods. But where foods compromise nutritional status they should be reduced or substituted. This is the case with caffeine, including drinks. Caffeine inhibits the absorption and conversion of certain minerals and trace elements, so it fights the aims of this eating plan. It also boosts adrenalin levels, which can aggravate mood swings and fluctuating blood sugar levels.

- **Stop**: Coffee; tea; cola; sarsaparilla.

- **Substitute**: Hot bouillon; herbal/fruit teas; diet tonic/bitter lemon/mineral water; diet ginger beer.

Eating Out and Take-away

Try not to eat out or have take-away for at least the first 3 weeks of your eating plan. Once you feel stabilised on your plan, the occasional restaurant meal or take-away should not cause any problems.

Unlike the other eating plans in this book, this one has few contra-indications to specific foods. The aim is not to avoid certain foods but to eat as healthily as possible. Once you have achieved a fairly healthy level of day-to-day eating, an infrequent blow-out is perfectly OK – though you may not feel great the morning after!

AT-A-GLANCE GUIDE TO STOP AND SUBSTITUTE FOODS

Stop – *Substitute*

Complex Carbohydrate Food Group

white bread – *brown bread*

Refined Carbohydrate Food Group

sugar – *sparing honey/fruit juice*
syrup – *sparing molasses*
biscuits – *rice cakes spread with cottage cheese*
cakes – *continental bread spread with diet fromage frais*
confectionery – *fruit*

Dairy Food Group

ice-cream – *frozen yoghurt*
chocolates – *bananas/see Snack Substitutes (p. 313)*
malted drinks – *skimmed milk with vanilla essence*
chocolate drinks/shakes – *yoghurt and fruit shakes*

Protein Food Group

spiced meats – *plain recipes*
fried meat and fish – *grilled/casseroled meat and fish*
salted nuts – *unsalted nuts*
junk food – *sandwiches*
Chinese take-away – *Greek take-away*
Indian take-away – *pizza*

Condiments

salt – *'low-salt'/herbs*
soy sauce – *sesame oil/home-made stock*
jam – *sparing honey*
commercial stock cubes – *home-made stock*
commercial sauce and gravy mix – *pan reductions*

Vegetable and Fruit Food Group

chips – *stir-fried parsnip and carrot sticks*
roast potatoes – *mashed/boiled/jacket potatoes*
tinned vegetables – *frozen vegetables*
canned fruit – *fresh fruit*
potato crisps – *olives/raw vegetable sticks*

Beverages

coffee – *hot bouillon*
tea – *herbal/fruit teas*
colas – *diet tonic/bitter lemon/mineral water*
sarsaparilla – *diet ginger beer*

SAMPLE SUBSTITUTION PROGRAMME

* Items marked with an asterisk are given in greater detail in the Snack Substitutes and Recipes sections (pp. 313, 324).

MONDAY

Breakfast

Normal 2 slices wholemeal toast with butter and marmalade; cereal with milk; sweetened orange juice; coffee with milk and sugar

Includes these Stop Foods Sweetened orange juice, sugar, coffee

Substitute 2 slices wholemeal toast with butter and marmalade; cereal with milk (no sugar); fresh squeezed orange juice; *hot lemon juice with honey

Elevenses

Normal biscuit; coffee with milk and sugar

Stop Biscuit, coffee, sugar

Substitute *plain oatcake; *hot lemon juice with honey

Lunch

Normal Bowl of soup; sausage roll and salad; apple; 1 glass wine

Stop None

Substitute None

Afternoon tea

Normal Piece of cake; cup of tea without sugar

Stop Cake, tea

Substitute *2 rice cakes spread with flavoured diet fromage frais; *hot spiced orange juice

Dinner

Normal Prawn cocktail with 2 slices brown bread; pasta in tomato sauce with courgettes
Stop None
Substitute None

TUESDAY

Breakfast

Normal I soft-boiled egg with 2 slices bread and butter; fresh orange juice; coffee
Stop Coffee
Substitute I soft-boiled egg with 2 slices bread and butter; fresh orange juice; *warm skimmed milk with vanilla essence

Elevenses

Normal American-style cookie; coffee
Stop Cookie, coffee
Substitute Orange; *hot bouillon

Lunch

Normal Fried chicken limb in breadcrumbs; chips; peas; individual portion fruit trifle; glass wine; coffee
Stop Fried chicken, chips, coffee
Substitute Plain grilled chicken limb; baked potato; peas; trifle; wine; sparkling mineral water

Afternoon tea

Normal Small bar of chocolate; tea
Stop Chocolate, tea
Substitute *Banana and Ryvita sandwich; *hot spiced orange juice

Dinner

Normal Packet of potato crisps; sausages; baked beans; 2 slices toast; flavoured jelly; 2 glasses wine; coffee; I chocolate truffle

Stop Potato crisps, sausages, coffee, truffle

Substitute Raw vegetable sticks; grilled continental sausage; baked beans; 2 slices toast; jelly; wine; *Piermont; tangerine

WEDNESDAY

Breakfast

Normal Cereal with milk; pancake with maple syrup; fresh squeezed orange juice; coffee

Stop Coffee

Substitute Cereal with milk; pancake with maple syrup (but not maple-flavoured syrup); fresh squeezed orange juice; *hot lemon juice with honey

Elevenses

Normal Shortcake biscuit; coffee

Stop Shortcake biscuit, coffee

Substitute *Rice cake spread with flavoured cottage cheese; *hot bouillon

Lunch

Normal Scotch egg salad; 2 slices brown bread; apple; wine; coffee

Stop Scotch egg, coffee

Substitute 2 slices ham; large continental salad; 2 slices brown bread; apple; wine; mineral water

Afternoon tea

Normal Snack bar; tea

Stop Snack bar, tea

Substitute *Oatcake; *hot bouillon

Dinner

Normal Bowl of soup; grilled lamb chop; spinach; mashed potato; tinned tomato; fresh unsugared fruit salad; coffee

Stop Coffee

Substitute Hot orange juice

THURSDAY

Breakfast

Normal 2 rashers of bacon and 1 fried egg on toast; fresh orange juice; coffee

Stop Coffee

Substitute 2 rashers of bacon and 1 fried egg on toast; fresh orange juice; *hot lemon juice with honey

Elevenses

Normal Chocolate digestive biscuit; coffee

Stop Biscuit, coffee

Substitute *2 Ryvitas spread with honey and flavoured cottage cheese; *hot spiced orange juice

Lunch

Normal Baked potato with cheese; salad; chocolate gâteau; coffee; Coca Cola

Stop Chocolate gâteau, Coca Cola, coffee

Substitute Baked potato with cheese; salad; *mashed banana with yoghurt and crumbled oatcake; sparkling mineral water; *warm milk with vanilla essence

Afternoon tea

Normal Egg sandwich; tea

Stop Tea

Substitute Egg sandwich; mineral water

Dinner

Normal Taramasalata with brown bread; commercially prepared cod and salmon fish pie; spinach; grilled tomatoes; 2 glasses wine; coffee; after-dinner mint

Stop Coffee, after-dinner mint

Substitute Taramasalata with brown bread; fish pie; spinach; grilled tomatoes; 2 glasses wine; mineral water; tangerine

FRIDAY

Breakfast

Normal Toast with jam; coffee

Stop Jam, coffee

Substitute Toast with Bovril; fresh orange juice

Elevenses

Normal Apple; coffee

Stop Coffee

Substitute Apple; *hot bouillon

Lunch

Normal Pork pie with chutney; tomato salad; 2 glasses wine; coffee

Stop Pork pie, coffee

Substitute Rice salad; tomato salad; 2 glasses wine; fresh orange juice

Afternoon tea

Normal Ginger biscuit; tea

Stop Ginger biscuit, tea

Substitute *Ryvita and flavoured cottage cheese; *hot lemon juice with honey

Dinner

Normal 3 measures spirit; Chinese take-away; 2 glasses wine; coffee; mint

Stop Chinese take-away, coffee, mint

Substitute 3 measures spirit (if you must); Greek take-away; 2 glasses wine; mineral water; orange quarters

SATURDAY

Breakfast

Normal I slice toast; coffee

Stop Coffee

Substitute I slice toast; orange juice

Elevenses

Normal Doughnut; coffee

Stop Doughnut, coffee

Substitute Egg custard tart; orange juice

Lunch

Normal Pub lunch of bread, cheese, chutney, salad, chips; ½ pint shandy

Stop Chips

Substitute Pub lunch of bread, cheese, chutney, salad, extra salad; ½ pint shandy

Afternoon tea

Normal Cake; tea

Stop Cake, tea

Substitute Honey and cottage cheese sandwiches made with soda bread; *hot lemon juice with honey

Dinner

Normal 2 measures spirit; avocado filled with prawns; steak; peas; baked potato; grilled tomatoes and mushrooms; ice-cream; 3 glasses wine

Stop None

Substitute None

SUNDAY

Breakfast

Normal Bacon; sausage; fried bread; grilled tomatoes; orange juice; coffee

Stop Sausage, coffee

Substitute Bacon; grilled continental sausage slices; fried bread; grilled tomatoes; fresh squeezed orange juice; mineral water

No elevenses today

Lunch

Normal 2 measures spirit; roast pork; mashed potato; cabbage; peas; gravy; apple pie with cream; coffee

Stop Coffee
Substitute 2 measures spirit; roast pork; mashed potato; cabbage; peas; gravy; apple pie with cream; *warm skimmed milk with vanilla essence

Afternoon tea

Normal Biscuit; tea
Stop Biscuit, tea
Substitute 1 slice toasted soda bread with honey; *hot spiced orange juice

Dinner

Normal Spanish omelette; salad; bread; cheese; celery; 2 glasses wine
Stop None
Substitute None

WHAT NEXT?

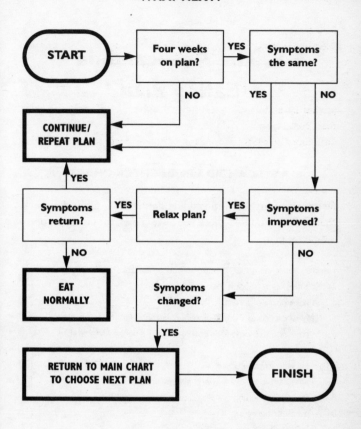

8. The Anti-candida Eating Plan

ANTI-CANDIDA PLAN CHECK CHART

Before you start the Anti-candida Eating Plan, fill in the check chart below to double-check you have chosen the most appropriate eating plan.

1. My abdomen is taut, bloated and uncomfortable below the waist. ☐
2. I suffer from trapped gas. ☐
3. I have bouts of thrush. ☐
4. My whole lower body is out of proportion with my top half. ☐
5. I have noticed some foods make me more uncomfortable than others. ☐
6. I have an irritable bowel. ☐
7. I am not overfat everywhere, just my abdomen. ☐
8. I feel very tired and congested on waking. ☐
9. I'm rather depressed. ☐
10. I have outbreaks of sore, flaking skin. ☐

Ticks KEY

0–3   Candida overgrowth is unlikely to be your main problem. Return to the flow chart and try to be more precise in your answers.

4–8   Candida is almost certainly your nutrition problem and the Anti-candida Eating Plan is likely to be a revelation to you.

9–10   Candida could still be your problem, but if you answered Yes to 4, you should start by looking at the Low-fat Eating Plan (p. 74) first. If

you answered Yes to 9, you need to ask yourself why you are
depressed. It could be that the Low-sugar or Menstrual Syndrome
Eating Plans (pp. 97, 181) might be better for you.

NOTE: Foods containing yeast – bread, blue cheeses, Marmite,
etc. – are most likely to upset candida sufferers.

WELCOME TO THE ANTI-CANDIDA EATING PLAN

This is the diet that's going to banish those bloated belly blues for
ever. Follow this path and you never need suffer an uncomfortable, distended abdomen again. Your tummy will become
flat and flexible – not rounded and taut.

You'll feel bright and breezy. Your digestion will improve and
your energy levels will go up. The familiar 'morning-after feeling'
of a heavy, squelchy tummy, gas and indigestion will gradually
disappear. Just imagine being able to forget that cloggy, bulky-
insides sensation and its depressing way of slowing you down.

Of all the different eating plans in this book, this is the one
closest to my heart – or should that be tummy? – because it
solves a problem that has driven most of us to give up hope. It's
that depressing bit of human body between waist and hips that
seems to swell and grow out of all proportion, determinedly
becoming the centre of your own and, you fear, everybody else's
attention.

If you wear trousers it looks as if your son has hidden his
football in them. Skirts betray you by creasing above and below
your tummy, allowing the unwelcome bulge complete freedom
to express itself. Only our old favourite, the stylishly baggy hip-
length sweater, is an ally in the campaign of concealment. And
the bloated tummy is uncomfortable too. It isn't just the
sensation of clothes restricting you. There are the inner problems
associated with it – poor digestion, gas, the feeling of being
waterlogged.

The worst of it is that the billow seems to be unbeatable. Conventional dieting merely makes it look more pronounced, as the rest of your body slims away to show it up more clearly. I've worked with super-slim fashion models whose skeleton-thin arms hugged their tummies but failed to cover up abdomens just as swollen as the rest of us.

Even endlessly repeated stomach exercises are of only limited help. They do produce a marvellous band of muscle over the top but all that does is help you pull in the billow – it doesn't get rid of it. This is because for most of us our swollen abdomen is not caused by excess fat at all. In women who are not especially obese – women who don't carry rolls of flesh elsewhere on their bodies – a sticky-out tummy is not caused by fat at all.

So what does cause this unwelcome protuberance? Bloating, not fat, is the cause. Let's start by enjoying this wonderful discovery. It's not fat! Hurray! No more guilt-ridden attempts to eat even less today than we did yesterday. Overeating is not the cause! No, candida is the cause. But what on earth is candida?

Candida albicans, to give the annoying stuff its full title, is a yeast-like fungus which every human being carries in their body from birth. It lives mainly in the bowel, but like other fungus it does have the ability to spread in extreme cases to other parts of the body. Nutritionists believe that as many as a third of us suffer from the effects of a mild degree of candida overgrowth. So when you are next in the changing-room at the gym and you notice how many of you take greater pains to conceal your bellies than any other part of your anatomy – just think, 33 per cent of us are probably fighting the candida battle. Doctors recognise candida officially as the micro-organism which we call 'thrush' – an unpleasant yeasty invasion of the vagina which causes a smelly discharge and itching. It can also be passed into the urinary system and cause cystitis.

The other, less widely recognised, effect of candida is the damage it can do to your digestive system. The candida in your digestive system is what we are concerned with here. It is what causes the bloating and distension which many of us have got to know too well for comfort. Candida behaves like other familiar yeasts in that it feeds itself through fermentation. Just as in making champagne, it eats sugar, metabolises it, grows and gives off fizzy gas – except that the result is not as nice as champagne at all.

The fermentation gases produce the most obvious problem – bloating – and often excess wind. Gradually, too, the body's ability to digest may be impaired, resulting in the combination of diarrhoea and constipation often vaguely titled 'irritable bowel'. The sheer bulk of the organism in the bowel may also increase enough to be a problem, causing the digestion to slow down and retain fluid. This may sound surprising in something like a yeast, but did you know that your bowels normally carry around a 4 lb weight of healthy bacteria alone?

Many alternative health practitioners and nutritionists also believe that candida overgrowth can eventually release toxins into the bloodstream, creating allergies and general ill-health. This has yet to be recognised by mainstream medical practitioners, and until it is I am inclined not to be convinced. In the first exhilaration at discovering the true cause of a long-term and widespread problem like abdominal bloating there is too great a temptation to rush ahead and believe you have also found the cure for a whole range of other hard-to-diagnose problems. It is best to concentrate on the specific relationship between candida and bloating – which is, after all, the problem most of us are concerned about.

Mild candida overgrowth now seems to be such a widespread problem that it's no wonder a slimmers' survey recently showed that more women had a problem with a swollen stomach than with pear-shaped hips. Now that we know about candida, though, it's easy to overcome it. And that's exactly what this diet is here to help you do. Stick to the Anti-candida Eating Plan and you will be able to conquer this yeast which can do so much to make you feel uncomfortable.

Normally candida is not much of a problem. Competing with other 'good' organisms in our intestines, like the digestive bacteria, keeps it in line. But various events can change the balance in candida's favour, and that's when it starts to get on top. If you have taken long-term or repeated antibiotics the candida gets ahead because antibiotics kill bacteria – the good ones included – so the proportion of candida is allowed to overwhelm the proportion of good bacteria in your bowel.

Another opportunity for candida to multiply is when you are taking oral contraceptives (the Pill), because this creates a hormonal state which is seventh heaven to candida. This is why women on the Pill tend to suffer thrush quite often. Other favourable circumstances for the overgrowth of candida occur when you are run down for some reason, so that the good bacteria in your body are busy fighting off infection rather than triumphing in the anti-candida battle.

Another very important reason for candida overgrowth is poor nutrition. Like any other yeast, candida thrives on sugar in whatever form, and modern refined diets tend to be comparatively high in sugar. Nutritionists and doctors believe this is why overgrowth of candida, or candidiasis as it's known medically, appears to be on the increase.

Although men do suffer from candida, and increasingly so, it is more often a female problem, due to hormones, contraception and the greater ease with which candida can move from bowel to urinary system in women because of the female anatomy. If candida invasion becomes so severe that you suffer chronic thrush or other serious symptoms, doctors can prescribe an anti-fungicide (Nystatin and Canestan are the most well known), but for most of us, the simple anti-candida diet will be all we need to restore our body to perfect functioning.

Read on now to discover how the Anti-candida Eating Plan works and how to put it into action and make it a part of your life. The aim of the diet is to starve the candida to death by depriving it of the sugars and sugar-containing carbohydrates from which it feeds. It's a simple diet that only requires you to give up certain foods – those that candida thrives on – and so that you don't starve to death along with the candida there is a whole range of replacement foods you can substitute instead.

HOW IT WORKS

Take heart! Being on a special diet doesn't mean you are fat. And there's more good news: being on the anti-candida programme won't force you into punishing months of self-sacrifice.

As we've discovered, candida overgrowth, not general fatness, is the cause of your sticking-out abdomen. So the Anti-candida Eating Plan is a specific, tailor-made plan designed to attack your candida alone. Because you don't have an overfat problem you don't need to count calories or reduce the fat in your diet. The ironic thing is that you could binge all day on those 'forbidden fatties' like crisps, peanuts and cheese, and it wouldn't make your candida worse at all.

This diet will meet your own personal needs – so there'll be no more plugging on with the misery of low-calorie regimes which do nothing for your abdomen and leave you so hungry you eventually break down and reach for the cake tin. In fact being forced to dive into the cake tin is exactly the worst thing that could happen to a candida sufferer. More than anything else candida thrives on sugar, so cakes will keep it growing and multiplying.

As we have discovered, candida is a yeast, and like all yeasts it needs sugar to live. So the aim of the Anti-candida Eating Plan is to starve candida to death and then encourage all the good bacteria in your body to take the opportunity to multiply without competition. Nutritionists call this 'bowel management', which is just a medical name for following the diet that is right for you.

To starve the candida all we need to do is deprive it of sugar. It's as simple as that. That means cutting sugar right out of your diet. It is amazing how big a part sugar plays in most people's diets – even if you don't take sugar in tea and coffee or sprinkle it on food, there are so many products which contain hidden sugar that it can be very hard to eradicate it completely from your diet. Did you know tomato ketchup is full of sugar? Everybody realises chocolate and biscuits are full of sugar – but tinned vegetables? Convenience meals? Sausages?! From now onwards you are going to have to become a real label-reader when you are doing your supermarket shopping.

Looking at the full list of what contains sugar can be depressing. Even healthy fruit is stacked full of natural, unrefined sugar. It looks as if it might mean living on gruel and water.

Have courage! The Anti-candida Eating Plan is here to help you. Instead of simply forbidding various foods, the diet works by substitution. For every food you must stop eating because of your candida, there's an alternative that you can eat to give yourself the same sort of satisfaction. So in the Anti-candida Eating Plan you'll find a whole list of non-sugar alternatives to chocolate, designed to give you as nearly as possible the same sort of satisfaction.

There's no point pretending, as most diets do, that we are never going to want – no, need – another bar of chocolate as long as we live. We are, that's that. When that need arrives, some of the time we will be disciplined enough to overcome it completely. Some of the time we will just have to give in – but most of the time we'll be between the two, that is, we'd quite like some chocolate but if there was something almost as good that we could think of it would probably do.

There are times when you will succumb to a stop food, but if we can reduce the percentage of these times as far as possible it will make the chances of success in the anti-candida programme far higher. This is what tennis players call 'hitting the percentage shots'. They avoid playing strokes that could be outright winners, but are much more difficult to pull off, and instead stick to the ones that are much easier to play and will keep them in the game – they may not help them win, but they will certainly prevent them losing. When you are in a tough spot, the 'percentage game' is the one to play.

To show you how the stop/substitute theory works on a day-to-day basis I have included a sample of what your week's eating probably is at the moment, with the foods you can stop and substitute to put you right on course with the Anti-candida Eating Plan shown alongside (see p. 250). This way you can see how minimal changes to your current eating will put you on the anti-candida programme.

It has always irritated me to read conventional diet books and see that they make absolutely no concessions to your existing pattern of eating and lifestyle. The diet writers seem not to know of the existence of pub lunches, Chinese take-aways, grisly canteen food and all the things people really do eat in their daily lives. I've taken the revolutionary, but obvious, step of actually basing the Anti-candida Eating Plan on a real person's eating habits. Simple, isn't it? If only they could have thought of it before.

The plan sticks as closely as possible to what you are likely to be eating anyway – including canteen food and Chinese take-away – and shows you how to modify that slightly by substituting certain foods. There are one or two foods which won't be available in your canteen, but you can easily bring these in to work with you or pop out to buy them from a nearby supermarket or delicatessen. If you work full-time at home as a mother it will be simpler for you because you can be your own canteen and can shop more easily.

Unfortunately, sugar is not the only thing which has to be cut out to beat candida. It is also important to stop eating yeast products as well. The reason for this is that the overgrowth of candida in your system is likely to have sensitised you to yeast. Because your body is already overloaded with one yeast – candida – adding more in the shape of bread yeast or alcohol yeast is likely to make your symptoms worse. The food yeasts won't actually feed your candida or help it grow, but they will act in the same way as candida to contribute to your bloating problems.

Again, yeast appears in more foods than you would imagine. Apart from bread it appears in the process of making alcohol, malt vinegar, even doughnuts and crumpets. Luckily many candida sufferers find that after sticking to the Anti-candida Eating Plan for a month or so their candida has decreased sufficiently for them to be able to eat one or two yeast products without any problem.

Bread, however, seems not to be one of the products that can easily be re-introduced into the diet. Yeast is obviously one reason for this, and the problem is easily solved by sticking to unproved, non-yeast breads like soda bread. However, there are other problems with bread. One is that is it very easily digested by the body into sugar. Just put a piece of bread in your mouth and keep sucking it without swallowing. Soon it will taste quite sweet – this is because your body is already partially digesting it into the very sugar which will feed your candida. Another problem is that most bread is made with wheat, and candida sufferers seem especially sensitive to wheat – this may be because of the active wheatgerm present in it.

So bread is a stop food for three reasons – yeast, sugar and wheat. In time you may find you can reintroduce some wheat products into your diet. Do so gradually and note how you react. You'll notice Ryvita listed as a substitute for bread on many occasions. Theoretically it is not ideal because it contains malt, but many different dieticians have found that it is remarkably well tolerated by candida sufferers. Ultimately only you can tell what works best for you.

The Anti-candida Eating Plan is not particularly low-fat or low-calorie. Like all the other diets in this book it is a 'horses for courses' diet which works on the principle that different dieters need different diets. But you must remember too that this may not always be the *same* different diet. As I explained in the introduction (p. 3), you may need to transfer from one diet to another as your dietary needs change. If you feel you have solved both problems, eat as you like until you feel any symptoms returning and then go back to whichever diet you find more appropriate.

For example, you may have started by following the Low-fat Eating Plan for 2 months to lose general overfat on your body. Only now that you have lost your all-over fat has your bloated abdomen problem become noticeable, so you have moved on to the Anti-candida Eating Plan. If you start to regain fat after a couple of months on the Anti-candida Eating Plan (very unlikely, since there is so little sugar in the diet), spend 2 weeks on the Low-fat Eating Plan before returning to the anti-candida plan.

It is possible to work on both a candida and an overfat problem at the same time, because the diets do not contradict each other. To do this just stop all the foods on both stop lists, and also stop any substitutes which appear on one of the stop lists. Any food not mentioned on any list can be eaten as much as you like. But if you find it very hard to stick to the combined diet, go back to just the one that suits you best.

Now is the time to get started on your Anti-candida Eating Plan. Read the rest of the diet carefully. The next section is a list of notes on exactly how to use it – if in doubt, copy them out and keep them handy.

STEP-BY-STEP GUIDE TO THE ANTI-CANDIDA PLAN

1 Read all sections of the diet carefully.

2 Learn what the stop foods are and why you must stop them.

3 Get familiar with all the substitutes and where to buy them.

4 Go through the week-long sample eating programme and work out how it will fit into your lifestyle.

5 If you are at all uncertain you can decide to follow the sample eating programme exactly for a week until you get the hang of things.

6 Learn how to make the snack substitutes.

7 Make a copy of the glance guide to stop and substitute foods.

8 Take the glance guide shopping with you to make sure you are stocking up on the right foods.

9 Remember that any food not mentioned as a stop food can be eaten whenever you like.

10 Note which drinks are to be stopped.

11 Eat plenty of fresh vegetables; these are not stop foods.

12 Follow the diet for at least 2 months before reviewing your symptoms and deciding whether to continue on it, change to another diet, or return to normal eating.

STOP, THINK, SUBSTITUTE

Which foods should I stop eating and what should I substitute?

Complex Carbohydrate Group

This food group covers what are usually known as the 'starchy' foods. These foods – like bread, wheat, pasta, potatoes – do contain sugar in them, but in its 'complex' unrefined form. The table sugar we use for sweetening is refined from two different complex carbohydrate foods – sugar beet and sugar cane.

Some of these complex carbohydrates also contain yeast. The most obvious of these is bread which has risen, or proved as we call it. The rising, as we all know, is caused by yeast. Bread which has no yeast is often known as unleavened. Wheat on its own also has a fungal content in its germ, the wheatgerm.

Not all complex carbohydrates feed candida. Nutritionists have found that wheat and risen bread are the two which encourage candida most, while others like potatoes and oat flakes do not seem to feed candida.

You only need to give up eating the complex carbohydrates listed below, and you can replace those with the substitutes listed, or just go on eating any other starchy foods which have not been mentioned – including chips!

- **Stop:** Risen/proved bread whether brown or white; Greek pitta bread; all kinds of pasta; wheat and wheat products; barley.

- **Substitute:** Soda bread, known as Scofa and available at supermarkets and bread shops; rice cakes, round crispbreads made out of puffed rice and available at major supermarkets and health stores in many different varieties; brown rice; beans and pulses (such as kidney beans and split peas); flaked oats and flaked rye, available from health stores and some supermarkets with health sections; and of course, potatoes.

Refined Carbohydrate Group

These are foods in which sugar is present in its refined state. Candida thrives on these foods, which are generally reckoned to be bad for all of us anyway. They are fattening because they contain lots of extra 'empty' sugar calories which have no other nutritional value in terms of the protein, vitamins and minerals the body needs. Some of the foods on the list – such as doughnuts and wine – also contain yeast, which is an extra blow to a digestion already trying to fight off an overload of candida yeast.

All refined carbohydrates – including cakes, chocolate and many convenience foods – are on the stop list for candida sufferers and the bad news is that there is no direct substitute within the group. If you think about it you couldn't really expect there to be – after all, what else will really do when what you crave is a chunk of chocolate? But these foods must be cut out if we are to starve that candida. Luckily in the years I have spent evolving the Anti-candida Eating Plan I have come up with lots of substitutes which are nearly as nice, even though they aren't quite the same. Most of them are so delicious, though, that after a while you'll forget about cakes.

Chocolate and biscuit lovers will have a slight problem at first. Chocolate especially has what food marketing experts call 'mouth appeal'. That means it is particularly satisfying and soothing while it is actually in the mouth. Very few foods possess this quality, and it is quite interesting to realise that when food manufacturers are creating new products they are always trying to invent something with the same 'mouth appeal'. Apparently it is the combination of the lactic acid available from the chocolate's dairy content, the texture of the cocoa, and the sweetness of the sugar which gives the dark little devil its terrible irresistibility.

But where can we find 'mouth appeal' outside chocolate? Dairy products generally can provide an element of it (just think of cream), and we are very lucky that there is one dairy product which is a positive ally in the anti-candida campaign. Yoghurt contains bacteria which are the right ones for your digestive system and can help displace the candida now flourishing in it. There are lots of very good yoghurts now that do not contain sugar but do contain the good bacteria, usually known as 'bifidus active' (often shortened to BA) or 'lactobacillus actifus'. Take a wander along your local supermarket's yoghurt counter and choose yourself a thick, creamy plain one and a flavoured one (check the label to make sure there is no sugar in it). At home, experiment – try it on its own, or with fruit, or with honey, or spread on oatcakes and rice cakes.

Not quite chocolate, it has to be admitted, but it does help ease the craving. Go on experimenting with different permitted combinations until you get as close as you can to that supreme chocolatey satisfaction!

Another good source of 'mouth appeal' is the banana. It has a good combination of texture and sweetness even if it lacks a chocolatey bite. Bananas are also extremely nutritious, and good providers of potassium, a trace element which can help prevent cravings. A mashed banana with creamy yoghurt often does the trick for me when what I would really like is two cubes of Cadbury's Dairy Milk. Or if it's something biscuity you desire, try sandwiching your banana between two Ryvitas. Not the real thing, I'm afraid, but close.

Table sugar itself you will have to give up. I use honey as a substitute. Honey too is a refined carbohydrate (the bees have done the refining for us), and it is nutritionally very similar indeed to sugar. Yet I have found that it does not seem to encourage candida anything like as much as table sugar, though some nutritionists disagree with me about this and the answer may be that one tends to use less honey than sugar and so those with only mild candida are less affected by it. You will have to experiment for yourself to see if you can tolerate honey; if not, cut it out too.

Some of the substitutes listed and marked with an asterisk have special recipes or purchasing details and you will find these detailed in the Snack Substitute section of the diet (p. 313).

- **Stop**: Cakes, biscuits, doughnuts, pâtisserie, sweet or wheat-based breakfast cereals; sugar; syrup; chocolates; wine (you may be able to tolerate certain other alcohols –

experiment); ice-cream; commercial puddings including sugar, yeast or wheat (read the label); sweets; convenience foods whether sweet or savoury if including sugar, yeast or wheat (read, read, read the label – never assume).

- **Substitute**: Soda bread, rice cakes or Ryvitas spread with honey or cottage cheese or fromage frais; oatcakes; breakfast cereals without sugar or wheat (read the label); home-made cream and fruit puddings; flavoured 'diet' yoghurts; plain yoghurt – especially any marked 'live' or 'bifidus active' or 'BA', as these contain helpful bacteria which can attack candida; fresh fruit without its peel and without any sign of mould; bananas (one of the few fruits with sufficient 'mouth appeal' to substitute for chocolate).

Protein Group

Few candida sufferers find meat and fish worsen their condition. These are the main providers of protein in our diet, and fortunately they do not contain sufficient sugars or yeast for the candida to feed from. Some nutritionists believe that if there is considerable candida overgrowth the digestion of meat can be impaired, but I have not found this.

Only commercially prepared meat products need worry most candida sufferers. English sausages contain bread and other meat products may contain sugar and pastry. Read the labels carefully and avoid any convenience food of this type. Continental sausages are usually 100 per cent meat and make an enjoyable substitute.

- **Stop**: Commercial meat products; sausages; pies; convenience meals.

- **Substitute**: Fresh home-made foods; fish products; continental sausages and dry-cured meats.

Vegetable and Fruit Group

Very few of the vegetable group cause any problems for candida sufferers. The basic rule is to eat plenty of fresh green vegetables and salads, as these are excellent health promoters and will help improve irritable bowel syndrome associated with candida.

Sauerkraut and pickles are fermented vegetables and as such contain yeast, which may well cause a candida-sensitised bowel to react badly. Mushrooms too, as fungi, may have a similar effect, but in fact many candida sufferers find they can manage mushrooms perfectly easily, particularly after they have been on the anti-candida programme for a while.

Tinned vegetables such as baked beans need checking carefully, as they often contain sugar, but the low-sugar versions seem generally acceptable, even though they often contain quite a high level of fruit sugar.

If you do find problems with the foods I have mentioned it is not a major difficulty because there are so many other interesting vegetables which you can eat instead. Any vegetable not mentioned in the stop list should be considered perfectly OK.

- **Stop**: Sauerkraut; pickles; tinned beans, etc.; mushrooms.

- **Substitute**: Shredded fresh cabbage; sliced cucumber with mint; home-cooked beans in tomato purée; chopped capsicums (green peppers); onions.

There is a lot of disagreement among nutritionists about how safe the fruit group of foods is for candida sufferers. The problem is that all fruits contain quite a high amount of sugar, as you would expect because they taste sweet. Although it is unrefined sugar when we eat it, the sugar rapidly becomes nutritionally very similar to refined sugar as our body begins to digest it.

So theoretically the sugar in fruit should provide the candida with food. In practice, though, the sugar in most fruit is diluted by the fruit's water content, so your body can extract less 'refined' sugar per piece of fruit that you eat than it can per spoonful of table sugar. Of course, if you were able to eat 20 oranges at a sitting you might well end up ingesting (taking in) a lot of sugar. But fortunately fruit is not the sort of thing you eat in twenties (unlike chocolates).

This is one of the reasons why dried fruit is on the stop list. Without its water content to bulk it out, dilute the sugar, and prevent you eating enormous quantities of it, you may well eat enough dried fruit to gain a substantial amount of sugar. Another problem with fruit is that it deteriorates quickly, and as it deteriorates moulds and fungi grow on it (not always visibly) to which a candida-sensitised digestion may react badly.

So those fruits which you always peel – oranges, tangerines, bananas – can be eaten in any amount. Apples, grapes, etc., generally eaten with the peel on, should be avoided at first. Later you can reintroduce them and watch out for any adverse reactions.

Fruit juices should be freshly squeezed and not sweetened. Sparkling apple juices seem to be fairly acceptable if not sweetened – especially good are those by Piermont, from supermarkets and many off-licences.

- **Stop**: Dried fruit, raisins, grapes, apples, dates, sweetened fruit juices.

- **Substitute**: Fresh fruit, chopped fresh fruit; nuts, especially unroasted almonds; olives; oranges; tangerines; fresh squeezed juices.

Dairy Group

For those trying to lose fat, giving up the dairy group foods is one of the greatest sacrifices, but the good news for anti-candida dieters is that dairy foods can be your biggest allies.

As we have already discussed, eating live unsweetened yoghurt is a great weapon in the anti-candida campaign. Equally helpful is the fact that cream, cream cheese and most ordinary cheese is perfectly allowable on the programme. So on those days when you simply must have something naughty but nice, lashings of cream cheese or a generous helping of clotted cream on your strawberries is perfectly OK.

I bet you never thought you'd read a diet which allowed double cream? But forbidden food is always the most tempting, so just to add a little spice I'll remind you that if you have had a tendency to put on fat in the past – for example if you have come on to this diet plan after succeeding on the Low-fat Eating Plan – you should try to save the whipped cream only for times when you really crave something special.

Some candida sufferers find they have to give up blue cheeses and ripe runny cheeses (like Camembert and Brie) because the mould content worsens their candida sensitivity. I think it is wise to exclude these cheeses to begin with and only reintroduce them into your diet occasionally if you get no adverse reaction to them.

Sweetened dairy foods and drinks like milk shakes and hot malted drinks are on the stop list, but there are a good variety of substitutes for these which are listed under Snack Substitutes (p. 313).

- **Stop**: Blue, ripe cheeses; malted drinks; milk shakes.

- **Substitute**: Plain hard cheeses; processed cheeses; yoghurt; yoghurt drinks; plain milk drinks.

Condiments

This group is not a food group in nutritional terms, but needs to be included because modern diets have a very high level of condiment content. Condiments are the dressings, seasonings and extras that we add to our foods to make them exciting. Often we only need them because over-processing has made them too bland, or to cover up unpleasant tastes in 'junk' food – try eating a sausage without tomato ketchup and then try eating a good fillet steak with tomato ketchup and you'll see what I mean.

Condiments are the invisible problem for many candida sufferers because they contain hidden sugars and yeasts, but since they are not regarded as a major part of the diet they are easily forgotten. Where many a low-fat or low-calorie dieter has fallen back on ketchups, vinegars and chutneys as an easy way of pepping up a boring diet, the anti-candida dieter must do the exact opposite. Vinegar, ketchup, chutney and Marmite contain yeasts and sugars which the anti-candida dieter must avoid. But luckily few main foodstuffs are forbidden, even if quite fatty, so the best thing is to enjoy the natural taste of good foods.

Until your tastebuds adjust you may need to use substitutes. I have given Bovril as a substitute for Marmite. Both of these do contain yeast, but for some reason Bovril does not seem to have such an adverse effect. If you find that it does, then stop Bovril as well as Marmite and rediscover the taste of good old butter instead.

- **Stop**: Marmite, vinegar, chutney, barley/malted sweetener, jam, ketchup.

- **Substitute**: Bovril (if satisfactory); lemon juice; savoury yoghurt or cottage cheese dips; honey; tomato purée or mushroom purée.

Beverages

Wine is made by a fermentation process similar to what is already going on in a candida sufferer's intestine. It does not make sense to add to this!

In fact, nutritionists believe that yeast products like wine do not actually worsen the candida condition but that a sufferer's body becomes so overloaded with yeasts that it becomes highly sensitised and intolerant to all yeasts. So while wine and other yeast products may not make the candida worse, they will make you *feel* worse – more bloated and less healthy.

It's a good idea to give up alcohol entirely, if you can, for at least 4 weeks. If not, at least give up wine and cut your intake of spirits to no more than one measure per day. Beer contains both yeast and malt, so should be given up completely.

Throughout your anti-candida dieting, if in doubt what to drink, have mineral water or fruit juice. Coffee and tea do not seem to be a problem for candida sufferers as long as they are taken without sugar. There are plenty of substitutes for other malted drinks and shakes, and recipes for these can be found in the Snack Substitutes section (p. 313).

Fizzy drinks like Coke, Pepsi, Fanta, etc. follow the normal rules of the Anti-candida Eating Plan – that is, if they contain sugar (and original Coke contains quite a few spoonfuls) you must stop them. Diet drinks not containing sugar are OK, but I do recommend that you avoid them as much as possible because they are very gassy and since this is already a problem for you it is not a good idea to take in extra fizz!

- **Stop**: Wine, too much alcohol, fizzy soft drinks, malted drinks and shakes.

- **Substitute**: Mineral water, Piermont (a flavoured mineral water available in supermarkets and off-licences), diet soft drinks (occasionally), home-made shakes and yoghurt drinks.

Junk Foods and Take-aways

I am not going to pretend that people on diets, whatever sort of diets, do not succumb to the lure of junk food and take-aways on Friday and Saturday nights. After a week of newshounding I would collapse gratefully in front of an enormous Chinese take-away on more Saturday nights than I care to admit. The good news for anti-candida dieters is that take-aways as such are not a major problem.

When choosing your junk food or take-away, use your common sense and try to stick as far as possible to the general rules of the Anti-candida Eating Plan, that is, avoid sugar or yeast. This means that a Big Mac is off limits because of the sesame bun, even though the burger itself (and the chips!) are OK. Traditional English fish and chips are fine provided you lay off the malt vinegar.

Greek take-away is not bad, but try to cut out the pitta bread if you can. Pizza topping is fine, but you may find the doughy pizza base does contribute to bloating and for this reason I cut down on it or avoid it altogether.

Chinese take-away is more or less unfathomable to a nutritionist – how on earth can you tell what the Chinese chef is up to with his wok – but the general rules can be applied. Obviously sweet dishes like sweet and sour prawns or crispy beef should be avoided. It is better too to choose rice rather than noodles. Everybody feels a bit bloated after a Chinese meal, but candida sufferers don't seem to find it any worse than anyone else, and the bloating disappears quite quickly , evidence that the Chinese food is not feeding the candida very efficiently. So I think you can be allowed the occasional Chinese treat.

In my experience Indian food is one of the best of all for candida sufferers. Perhaps this is because it is a cuisine originally designed for a hot, often damp, climate where beating yeasts and moulds was very important. Most Indian breads are made without yeasts and prove to be very acceptable to candida sufferers. Yoghurt is used a great deal in Indian recipes, and this too suits candida sufferers. Where low-fat dieters have to avoid Indian dishes like the plague because of the high-fat 'ghee' used in their preparation, I think the candida sufferer can tuck in fairly happily – unless the fat is starting to pile on, in which case it's time to switch over to the Low-fat Eating Plan for a while!

- **Stop:** Big Macs; pizzas; pitta bread; sweet Chinese dishes.

- **Substitute:** Traditional fish and chips; plainer Chinese dishes; Indian take-away.

AT-A-GLANCE GUIDE TO STOP AND SUBSTITUTE FOODS

Stop – *Substitute*

Complex Carbohydrate Food Group

risen bread – *soda bread/rice cakes*
pitta bread – *most crispbreads/matzo biscuits*
pasta – *brown rice/beans/pulses*
wheat – *flaked oats*
barley – *flaked rye*

sugar – *honey*
syrup – *cream/fresh squeezed orange juice*
chocolates – *banana/Ryvita banana sandwich*
alcohol/wine – *sparkling fruit juice*
ice-cream – *frozen yoghurt*
commercial puddings – *diet fruit fromage frais*
sweets – *fruit*
convenience foods – *home-made snacks*

Refined Carbohydrate Food Group

cakes – *soda bread with honey and cottage cheese*
biscuits – *oatcakes*
doughnuts – *rice cakes with honey*

Protein Food Group

commercial pies and meals – *home-made*
English-style sausages – *continental sausages*

Vegetable and Fruit Food Group

sauerkraut – *shredded fresh cabbage*
pickles – *sliced cucumber*
canned baked beans – *home-prepared beans in tomato*
mushrooms – *green capsicums/onions*
dried fruit – *chopped fresh fruit*
raisins – *flaked almonds*
grapes – *olives*
apples – *oranges*
dates – *tangerines*
sweetened fruit juice – *fresh squeezed orange juice*

Dairy Food Group

blue cheeses – *plain cheese*

chocolate drinks – *yoghurt and juice mix*
'ripe' cheeses, including Brie and Camembert – *processed cheese*
milk shakes – *milk and fruit purée*

Condiments

Marmite – *Bovril*
vinegar – *lemon juice*
chutney – *savoury yoghurt dip*
sweetener – *honey*
jam – *honey*

SAMPLE SUBSTITUTION PROGRAMME

* Items marked with an asterisk are given in greater detail in the Snack Substitutes and Recipes sections (pp. 313, 324).

MONDAY

Breakfast

Normal 2 slices wholemeal toast with butter and marmalade; cereal with milk; sweetened orange juice; coffee with milk and sugar

Includes these Stop Foods Wholemeal bread, marmalade, cereal, sweetened orange juice, sugar

Substitute 2 slices soda bread toast with butter and honey; pure oatflakes with milk; fresh squeezed orange juice; coffee with milk

Elevenses

Normal biscuit; coffee with milk and sugar

Stop Biscuit, sugar

Substitute *plain oatcake; coffee with milk

Lunch

Normal Bowl of soup; sausage roll and salad; apple; I glass wine

Stop Sausage roll, apple, wine

Substitute Bowl of soup; ham and salad; orange; sparkling mineral water

Afternoon tea

Normal Piece of cake; cup of tea without sugar

Stop Cake

Substitute *2 rice cakes spread with flavoured diet fromage frais; cup of tea

Dinner

Normal Prawn cocktail with 2 slices brown bread; pasta in tomato sauce with courgettes; ice-cream

Stop Brown bread, pasta, ice-cream

Substitute Prawn cocktail with 2 Ryvitas; *risotto with tomatoes and herbs; courgettes; *plain yoghurt mashed with frozen raspberries

TUESDAY

Breakfast

Normal I soft-boiled egg with 2 slices bread and butter; fresh orange juice; coffee

Stop Bread

Substitute I soft-boiled egg with 2 Ryvitas; fresh orange juice; coffee

Elevenses

Normal American-style cookie; coffee

Stop Cookie

Substitute Orange; coffee

Lunch

Normal Fried chicken limb in breadcrumbs; chips; peas; individual portion fruit trifle; 1 glass wine; coffee

Stop Breadcrumbs, trifle, wine

Substitute Plain chicken limb (or scrape off breadcrumbs); chips; peas; fruit salad with yoghurt; sparkling mineral water; coffee

Afternoon tea

Normal Small bar of chocolate; tea

Stop Chocolate

Substitute *Banana and Ryvita sandwich

Dinner

Normal Packet of potato crisps; sausages; baked beans; 2 slices toast; flavoured jelly; 2 glasses wine; coffee; 1 chocolate truffle

Stop Sausages, baked beans, toast, jelly, wine, truffle

Substitute Packet of potato crisps; grilled continental sausage; *home-cooked mixed pulses in fresh tomato sauce; 2 slices oven-warmed soda bread; portion plain creamy yoghurt sprinkled with honey and walnuts; *Piermont; coffee; tangerine

WEDNESDAY

Breakfast

Normal Cereal with milk; pancake with maple syrup; fresh squeezed orange juice; coffee

Stop Cereal, maple syrup

Substitute Oatflakes with milk and chopped banana; pancake with butter and honey; fresh squeezed orange juice; coffee

Elevenses

Normal Shortcake biscuit; coffee

Stop Shortcake biscuit

Substitute *Rice cake spread with flavoured cottage cheese; coffee

Lunch

Normal Scotch egg salad; 2 slices brown bread; apple; wine; coffee

Stop Scotch egg, brown bread, apple, wine

Substitute 2 slices smoked ham; large continental salad; 2 slices crispbread; orange; sparkling mineral water; coffee

Afternoon tea

Normal Snack bar; tea

Stop Snack bar

Substitute *Oatcake; tea

Dinner

Normal Bowl of soup; grilled lamb chop; spinach; mashed potato; tinned tomato; fresh unsugared fruit salad; coffee

Stop None

Substitute None

THURSDAY

Breakfast

Normal 2 rashers of bacon and 1 fried egg on toast; fresh orange juice; coffee

Stop Toast

Substitute 2 rashers of bacon and 1 fried egg on a thick slice of soda bread; fresh orange juice; coffee

Elevenses

Normal Chocolate digestive biscuit; coffee

Stop Biscuit

Substitute *2 Ryvitas spread with honey and flavoured cottage cheese; coffee

Lunch

Normal Baked potato with cheese; salad; chocolate gâteau; coffee; Coca Cola

Stop Chocolate gâteau, Coca Cola

Substitute Baked potato with cheese; salad; *mashed banana with yoghurt and crumbled oatcake; coffee; Diet Coke

Afternoon tea

Normal Egg sandwich; tea

Stop Bread

Substitute 2 slices Ryvita sandwiched round sliced egg and tomato; tea

Dinner

Normal Taramasalata with brown bread; commercially prepared cod and salmon fish pie; spinach; grilled tomatoes; ice-cream; 2 glasses wine; coffee; after-dinner mint

Stop Bread, commercially prepared meal (if ingredients list includes sugar, if not no need to substitute), ice-cream, wine, mint

Substitute Taramasalata with water biscuits; if fish pie contains sugar, then *home-made fish pie, otherwise don't worry; *frozen yoghurt; *Piermont; kiwi fruit

FRIDAY

Breakfast

Normal Toast with jam; coffee

Stop Toast, jam

Substitute *2 rice cakes spread with butter and honey; fresh orange juice; coffee

Elevenses

Normal Apple; coffee

Stop Apple

Substitute Banana; coffee

Lunch

Normal Pork pie with chutney; tomato salad; 2 glasses wine; coffee

Stop Pork pie, chutney, wine

Substitute Rice salad; tomato salad; fresh orange juice; coffee

Afternoon tea

Normal Ginger biscuit; tea

Stop Ginger biscuit

Substitute Ryvita and flavoured cottage cheese; tea

Dinner

Normal 3 measures spirit; Chinese take-away; 2 glasses wine; coffee; mint

Stop Any sweet or sweet and sour Chinese dishes, wine, mint

Substitute 3 measures spirit (if you must); Chinese take-away without dishes like sweet and sour pork or crispy beef; 2 glasses diet cola; coffee; orange quarters

SATURDAY

Breakfast

Normal 1 slice toast; coffee

Stop Toast

Substitute Orange segmented and garnished with roasted almonds; coffee; sparkling mineral water

Elevenses

Normal Doughnut; coffee

Stop Doughnut

Substitute Egg custard tart; coffee. While not completely sugar free at least the egg custard contains no yeast, and if you are out doing your weekend shopping a café is unlikely to provide rice cakes!

Lunch

Normal Pub lunch of bread, cheese, chutney, salad, chips; ½ pint shandy

Stop Bread, chutney, shandy

Substitute Pub lunch of gammon with pineapple; salad; chips; tomato juice or Diet Coke

Afternoon tea

Normal Cake; tea

Stop Cake

Substitute Honey and cottage cheese sandwiches made with soda bread; tea

Dinner

Normal 2 measures spirit; avocado filled with prawns; steak; peas; baked potato; grilled tomatoes and mushrooms; ice-cream; 3 glasses wine

Stop Ice-cream, wine

Substitute 2 measures spirit (it is Saturday after all); avocado filled with prawns; steak; peas; baked potato; grilled tomatoes and mushrooms; fresh fruit salad; sparkling mineral water

SUNDAY

Breakfast

Normal Bacon; sausage; fried bread; grilled tomatoes; orange juice; coffee

Stop Sausage, bread

Substitute Bacon; grilled continental sausage slices; toasted soda bread; grilled tomatoes; fresh squeezed orange juice; coffee

No elevenses today

Lunch

Normal 2 measures spirit; roast pork; mashed potato; cabbage; peas; gravy; apple pie with cream; coffee

Stop Apple pie

Substitute 2 measures spirit; roast pork; mashed potato; cabbage; peas; gravy; *stewed fruit (oranges, bananas, peeled sliced apples) with cream and a garnish of crumbled oatcake; coffee

Afternoon tea

Normal Biscuit; tea

Stop Biscuit

Substitute 1 slice toasted soda bread with honey; tea

Dinner

Normal Spanish omelette; salad; bread; cheese; celery; 2 glasses wine
Stop Bread, wine
Substitute Spanish omelette; salad; oven-warmed soda bread; cheese; celery;
*Piermont

WHAT NEXT?

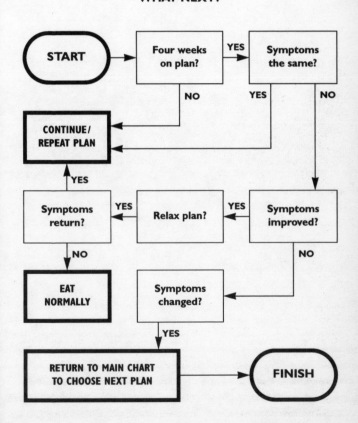

9. The Low-allergen Eating Plan

LOW-ALLERGEN EATING PLAN CHECK CHART

Before you start the Low-allergen Eating Plan, fill in the check chart below by ticking any Yes answers to double-check that you have chosen the most appropriate eating plan.

1. I have noticed I react badly to certain foods and/or environmental sources (e.g. cats give me a rash). ☐
2. I am asthmatic. ☐
3. I have eczema/related skin conditions. ☐
4. I often have a bloated stomach. ☐
5. I have frequent migraines. ☐
6. I have puffy, pudgy thighs. ☐
7. I am taking oral contraceptives. ☐
8. I eat a disproportionate amount of certain foods. ☐
9. My eyes are very sensitive to strong light. ☐
10. My symptoms are worse on a monthly cycle. ☐

Ticks KEY

0–3   If you have answered Yes to 2 or 3, you may very well have a food sensitivity or intolerance and it will be worth investigating this eating plan, even though you do not have other symptoms. But if these were not among the 0–3 to which you answered Yes, it is advisable to go back to the Eating Plans Map (pp. 12–13) and try for a closer diagnosis.

4–8   A food sensitivity/intolerance may well be at the root of your
          problems. Read the advice in this eating plan and try to find a
          sympathetic practitioner to help you explore your possible allergies
          (see addresses on pp. 337–8).

9–10 While you may indeed have a food intolerance, it is likely that other
          eating problems are more pressing. If you answered Yes to 6, look at
          the Low-fat Eating Plan check chart (p. 74). If you answered Yes to 7,
          it may be that oral contraception is not suitable for you. Discuss this
          with your family planning practitioner. If you answered Yes to 10, try
          the Menstrual Syndrome Eating Plan (p. 181) before returning to this
          eating plan if you do not achieve an improvement.

WHAT IS FOOD ALLERGY/INTOLERANCE?

When we read in the newspaper of someone who has died after
eating peanuts, or a friend has to refuse strawberries because she
reacts badly to them, we recognise these as cases of food allergy.
So does orthodox medicine. This form of acute food sensitivity
or intolerance is well known and accepted. It is called 'acute'
because the symptoms have a swift onset, causing suffering
which must be relieved immediately; once treated, however, the
symptoms disappear very quickly.

A chronic illness, by contrast, can have a slow (often barely
noticeable) onset of symptoms. The suffering caused can be
tolerated for long periods and the symptoms take a long time to
respond to treatment.

While acute food allergy is well accepted in orthodox
medicine, the concept of chronic food allergy is very recent and
not generally recognised. Chronic allergy can cause a wide range
of symptoms. One that many people are beginning to notice is
being overfat. Many people have discovered that simply by
omitting certain foods from their diet, rather than going on a
conventional slimming diet, they have been able to lose stubborn

fat that has resisted everything else. This is why, though still unorthodox, the concept of chronic food allergy is so exciting to anyone who suffers overfat problems.

Among the first major articles on the subject to appear in a recognised British medical publication was 'Food Allergy: fact or fiction?' by Dr Ronald Finn and Dr H. Newman, published in the *Lancet* in February 1978. Another milestone was the publication in 1984 of 'Food Intolerance and Food Allergy' by the Royal College of Physicians and the British Nutrition Foundation.

The initial shaping of the theory was that there might be certain foods which could cause some individuals to suffer chronic health problems and mood disorders. These foods or 'allergens' would not cause the sort of acute reaction so far accepted as allergy, but could contribute in a more complex way to problems including asthma, migraine, hyperactivity, etc. Certain chronic illnesses, like coeliac disease (a disease of the intestine caused by allergy to gluten), were already known to be connected with food intolerance, and the researchers wanted to spread the net wider to show that many types of illness resistant to other forms of treatment responded to dietary changes.

Among the theories put forward during the late 70s and early 80s was that artificial food colourings and additives could cause hyperactivity and health problems in children. At this time it was thought that many young children with digestive problems were intolerant of cow's milk, and this view is now seen as far less controversial.

Clinicians treating asthma, eczema and migraine also reported good results from manipulation of diet. So the idea of chronic intolerance of certain foods playing a part in recognised illness is now broadly accepted by orthodox medicine.

In the last decade, however, many researchers in the field of allergy have put forward the view that food intolerance is also implicated in a wide range of less well-quantifiable health problems. They associate food intolerance with many of the

vague disruptions of our well-being with which most of us are
familiar: indigestion; fatigue; constipation; bloatedness; poor
skin; aches and pains; rashes; moodiness; difficulty in weight
control.

This is the controversial area of food allergy practice.
Orthodox doctors quite rightly point out that such vague and
often trivial complaints cannot be tested in any controlled way.
They come under the category 'lack of well-being', which many
doctors feel is not really the province of medicine. The trouble is
that 'lack of well-being' can be caused by so many different
things – stress, depression, poor lifestyle, viral infection, as well
as genuine illness. 'Well-being' is also a totally subjective
phenomenon. Someone who has enjoyed good health throughout early adulthood will regard the ageing process as a loss of
well-being, while another person who has suffered illness at
various stages in their life will accept the same state of physical
fitness and health as complete well-being.

Some doctors think that in the West our expectations of well-
being are simply too high. Looking at the ethos in West Coast
America, where even wrinkles are regarded as unacceptable, one
is tempted to agree. Yet medical science has advanced so much in
the last century that most of us feel justified in assuming that it
will continue to contribute to improving our state of well-being.
In the past the infant mortality rate was far higher than it is
today. Pneumonia was a life-threatening illness. Today we
expect most illnesses to be curable; in the past people expected to
die from them.

So today perhaps we also have a right to expect maximum
well-being. If we are to succeed in this, though, the key will be to
take an active and positive role in creating good health. When we
suffer from a recognised illness we passively expect the doctor to
cure us with the minimum of commitment on our part. Give us
the tablet, we say, and we'll take it (as long as it's easy to
swallow).

The treatment of lack of well-being demands that we take a very different attitude. First we must realise that our well-being is our own responsibility, not the doctor's. Many doctors will do all they can to help you achieve well-being, but they can't be well for you.

The crucial first step is to identify as precisely as you can just what your lack of well-being is. Does it go on all the time? Does it have very obvious physical effects on you? The more of these certainties you can pin down, the better you and your doctor can help you.

Will food allergy/intolerance be one of the problems you discover? Orthodox medicine says that this still has not been proved likely. But anecdotal evidence (everyday experience) is increasingly showing that food intolerances and poor diet do indeed have an effect on well-being.

Typical is the laboratory in York which had been working for many years discovering the allergens in those who suffer from recognised allergic conditions. They found that once the specific allergen had been discovered and excluded from the diet, sufferers reported that not only had their obvious symptoms cleared up but they had also lost weight and generally felt better in every way.

Was this because the allergic condition had been depressing them and causing them to eat too much and feel generally poorly? Or was it because the allergen itself was causing the body to retain bulky fluid (making them overweight) and chemically depressing the nervous system? It is almost impossible to know.

Until many more research studies, stringently controlled, are carried out on those demonstrating only non-specific symptoms of lack of well-being, we cannot reach any firm conclusions. In the meantime, though, we can say that there are many people who have been able to lose weight and improve their general health greatly after excluding certain foods from their diet.

As you read through this chapter you will see that many of the food-related causes of lack of well-being have very specific signs.

Chronic chestiness and catarrh, for example, give the hint of a food allergy even if you do not suffer full-blown asthma. Some food sensitivities though, are believed to stem from 'masked allergens'. A masked allergen has no obvious effect on you. Indeed it is likely to be something you eat very, very frequently. Its effects only show under certain circumstances.

The major circumstance you are likely to come across is 'total overload'. This is when your immune system ceases to be able to cope with the allergen to which you are sensitive because so many other factors are already compromising the system. For example, you may drink coffee with no ill effects until you have a viral infection, when suddenly even the mere thought of it makes you sick. Or perhaps you have no problem with wine unless you are pre-menstrual. These are examples of other factors combining with a food sensitivity to tip the symptoms into the area of being noticeably unpleasant, sometimes acute.

Another circumstance which shows the effect of a masked allergen is its sudden withdrawal. This is similar to an addict going 'cold turkey'. While you are drinking your four or five cups of coffee a day you feel fine, but if for some reason coffee is no longer available you suddenly notice how awful you feel – headachy, dizzy, shivery, lack of concentration, aching bones. Occasionally you can overload on a masked allergen (rather like an overdose). If you suddenly have ten or twelve cups of coffee in a day instead of your usual four or five you will notice much the same reactions as if you had had none.

In fact, one of the easiest ways to spot a masked allergen is to look at any food to which you are really addicted. It's likely that this food is an allergen setting up a vicious circle of chemical reactions in your body. This works very much like an addiction to opium. When the food is consumed the body's chemical system reacts with unusual sensitivity, which at first means that the eater gets increased pleasure from the food. Naturally this leads to a desire to eat the food, but eventually it may be found that not eating the food causes withdrawal symptoms. After a period of time the saturation stage is reached, and at this point allergic reactions are felt – though the sufferer is unlikely to relate the symptoms to a food which he has enjoyed eating for some time.

As we have discovered, food allergy is a complex and ill-defined area. Follow the information in this chapter closely and you may be able to discover a food allergy and cure it single-handed. Alternatively, you may feel that you need help from a specialist (see addresses on pp. 337–8). However, in the excitement at finding a new possible cause of ill-health it is all too easy for converts to assume it applies to everyone. As you know, the whole principle of this book is that not every individual will have the same diagnosis. One of the reasons orthodox doctors are irritated by allergy specialists is because of their tendency to prescribe allergy treatment as a cure-all. It is not a cure-all. You may very well not have a food allergy. Remember, not everybody has a food allergy, so don't look for what isn't there.

If your overfat problem and any lack of well-being genuinely responds to allergy treatment, great. If not, don't pretend it does. Try something else. After all, there are ten other eating plans in this book.

MAIN ALLERGIC SYMPTOMS

The symptoms listed below very often lead to a clear-cut diagnosis of food/environmental allergy. In these cases orthodox medical thinking recognises the role of food/environmental intolerances to the extent that most clinicians now feel comfortable using the word 'allergy'.

Acute Reaction

Symptoms are marked and onset is rapid and requires urgent treatment on ingestion of food or contact with environmental source. Breathlessness, seizure, acute severe rash, pulse and heart rate changes, choking, muscular spasm. Can lead to death if not treated. The reaction most commonly referred to as allergy.

Asthma

Chronic breathing problems associated with collapsed lung, rashes and general ill-health. A key indicator of intolerance syndrome. Rarely present without other symptoms.

Eczema

Chronic skin problems often linked with asthma and other intolerance reactions. Because of the social problems triggered by eczema, depression and personality problems often ensue.

Migraine

Repeated acute headache attacks of varying duration associated with extreme local pain, vomiting, flashing lights, dizziness, nausea, muscular spasm and mood changes.

Coeliac Disease

A degenerative bowel condition linked with intolerance to gluten.

Failure to thrive

Condition of children where weight is not gained at a healthy rate, linked with general ill-health, mild disabilities, personality and learning disorders. May be caused by a complex set of factors now thought to include food intolerance, especially lactose sensitivity.

Vomiting

Immediate acute reaction to eating the allergen, e.g. oysters. Recovery generally fairly swift after stomach has been emptied.

SECONDARY ALLERGIC/INTOLERANCE SYMPTOMS

Orthodox clinicians currently do not generally regard the following symptoms as prima facie evidence of food or environmental allergy. Increasingly, though, they are being seen as contributory factors in a syndrome, and many more practitioners are now willing to consider looking at food/environment as possible causes. At this level, though, the phrase 'intolerance' or 'sensitivity' is felt to be more acceptable as an accurate reflection of the condition than 'allergy'.

Chronic Obesity
Only recently associated with food intolerance and still viewed as highly unorthodox. However, anecdotal evidence of weight loss following a low-allergen diet is rapidly increasing.

Chronic Catarrh
Despite apparent links with asthma, chronic catarrh is still little recognised as a health problem. Its implication in food intolerance has largely been discovered as a side effect by those following low-allergen diets for other reasons. Lactose and nicotine seem to be the main allergens.

Arthritis
Many sufferers report an improvement in their symptoms following dietary changes, and this is currently being researched with very positive early results.

Mood Changes
So hard to quantify that unless the changes are really acute they are unlikely to be an acceptable symptom. The placebo effect is very evident here and makes controlled trials very difficult.

Chronic Fatigue

Hard to quantify. The existence of a chronic fatigue syndrome has been posited by some researchers but is not widely accepted. However, anecdotal evidence suggests that food/environment intolerances may contribute to lack of well-being. Certainly the act of seeking any form of diagnosis and treatment may in itself commit the patient to fighting their fatigue whatever its cause.

Constipation

Obviously linked to dietary intake.

Fluid Retention

Most nutritionists now believe that many cases of fluid retention are caused by sensitivity to certain foods. Already intolerance of yeast is recognised as being involved in the fluid retention and bloating caused by candidiasis (see Anti-candida Eating Plan, p. 228).

Photosensitivity

Marked sensitivity to glare, e.g. head lamps at night, is regarded as a symptom by those practising in the allergy field.

Eye Problems

Asymmetric dilation of the pupils is often looked for by allergy practitioners, but it is also a symptom of other acute nervous disorders. If you have this problem, see your orthodox family doctor before visiting any other practitioners.

Neurotic Syndrome

Currently a very controversial area. The patient presents a complex of varying, often unquantifiable, symptoms, some of which may respond to treatment only to be replaced by other symptoms. Often associated with mood disorders. Conventional medicine tends to favour some form of psychiatric therapy. Allergy practitioners believe that food intolerances are implicated.

Failure to Respond to Treatment

Good diagnosticians work on an elimination principle. Basically this means regarding every possible cause as guilty until it is proved innocent. The diagnostician starts with the most dangerous possible cause of a symptom (even if it is also the most unlikely) and studies all the factors involved until he is sure it can be eliminated. Eventually he reaches a possible cause which cannot be eliminated, 'proved innocent', and this he treats. If the treatment is followed scrupulously by the patient but fails, it is likely that the diagnosis is wrong. Therefore the process of elimination must be started again. In this way clinicians sometimes arrive in the end at a food intolerance diagnosis – often their first experience of the diagnosis.

MAIN ALLERGEN GROUPS

A food, substance or environmental source (pollution, animals, etc.) which causes an allergic reaction is called an allergen. Certain foods are recognised as being more likely to cause a reaction than others. Seafood, for example, is well known as a common allergen. The main allergen groups are listed below. These are the ones that an allergy specialist will check for first.

Dairy

Cow's milk is the most common, along with cheese, butter and cow meat products. Often sufferers can tolerate some dairy products but not others. Medically known as the lactose group sensitivity.

Grains

Wheat and corn/maize are the main offenders. Some sufferers can still tolerate rye, oats, barley, etc. Coeliac disease is caused by an allergy to the gluten content of wheat and gluten products. Grain intolerance is known as gluten sensitivity.

Nicotine

Passive smokers are affected as badly or worse than smokers. The mere smell of cigarette smoke can trigger migraines in those intolerant of nicotine.

Alcohol

Wine is the main problem product in the group. This intolerance may be linked with yeast sensitivity (see the Anti-candida Eating Plan, p. 228). Grain distilled alcohols are likely to be problematic for grain sensitives.

Caffeine

A common trigger of migraine, though more rarely of general intolerance symptoms.

Chocolate

A common trigger of migraine. Generally a masked allergen. Its intolerance may be linked with its role as a factor in hypoglycaemic syndrome (see the Low-sugar Eating Plan, p. 97).

Sugar

Refined carbohydrates may be linked with allergy symptoms, but it is more likely that the problem is linked with hypoglycaemic syndrome (see the Low-sugar Eating Plan, p. 97).

Colourings

A well-known and now largely accepted cause of allergic symptoms, especially in children. Artificial colourings (coal tar, tartrazine, sunset yellow, etc.) are now less widely used in food products but can still cause allergic reactions if used in a non-food product, e.g. moisturiser, bubble bath, etc.

Additives

Many widely used additives, e.g. monosodium glutamate, can cause allergic reactions, as well as the better-known 'E' number additives which are now more closely regulated than in the past.

Environmental

Non-food, i.e. environmental factors, include the following: house dust mites (asthma); animals (asthma); man-made fibres (eczema); perfumes (asthma, eczema, migraine); out-gassing from plastic products (asthma, migraine); chemical treatments (asthma, eczema); diesel/petrol fumes (migraine); chlorine (migraine); household cleaning products (asthma, eczema, migraine).

Citrus

Oranges, citrus fruits generally, and citrus juices are often an allergen.

Eggs

Possibly associated with the gluten allergy group.

Pork Products

Sufferers are likely to find even the smell of pork upsetting.

Tap water

Recently becoming more evident, especially with increasing fluoridation of tap water.

STEP-BY-STEP GUIDE TO THE LOW ALLERGEN EATING PLAN

1   Read all sections of this chapter carefully.
2   Do you think you still have a food allergy?
3   Discuss your symptoms with your family doctor.
4   Is your doctor offering you satisfactory/appropriate treatment (whatever his diagnosis)? If yes, then work with him.
5   If your doctor is unhelpful but you are still convinced your problem is a food allergy continue with the plan.
6   Follow the weekly elimination programme.
7   Keep a diary of your symptoms.
8   Read all ingredient labels very carefully; if in doubt leave it out.
9   Start the reintroduction programme.
10 Note your symptoms.
11 Are your reactions very marked?
12 If yes, see an allergy practitioner (see addresses on pp. 337–8) and work with him.

WEEKLY ELIMINATION PROGRAMME

Method

- In the first week, exclude the first group mentioned. In the second week continue to exclude the first food and in addition exclude the second food. Continue this process until you have made all the exclusions. Do not reintroduce any food at this stage.
- Be extremely careful in your eliminations. You will have to read the label of every food product closely to make sure that it does not contain an ingredient that you are eliminating. Check over the section on reading labels on p. 16 before you start.

- At the end of each week, note any changes in your symptoms. Remember, you may get a delayed result from an elimination, so you will not be able to get an effective set of results until you have completed both the elimination and reintroduction programmes and compared notes.
- When you have finished the elimination programme, spend a further week with all the exclusions in place. This will give you time to stabilise before beginning the reintroductions.
- Reintroduce one food group at a time on a weekly basis, as shown in the reintroduction programme below.
- If you notice an extreme reaction to one of your reintroductions exclude it from your diet, but still continue on the programme of other reintroductions as normal. You may be sensitive to other foods.
- If you feel you have a conclusive result at the end of the two programmes, continue to exclude the foods to which you have decided you are sensitive. Other foods to which you have no reaction can be eaten regularly.
- If you find yourself so addicted to one particular food that you cannot persuade yourself to exclude it from your diet, suspect that you may be intolerant of it.
- You may not get a conclusive result at the end of your programmes. Food/environmental intolerance can be a complicated syndrome. The programmes test for the most common allergens, but you will probably need help from an allergen practitioner.

Elimination Programme

Week One – Dairy

Products eliminated Milk, butter, cheese, yoghurt, dairy products, low-fat spread, anything containing dairy.

Any changes in symptoms at end of week?

Week Two – Grains

Products eliminated Wheat, flour, bread, corn, corn oil, rye, oats, barley, rice, products containing grains.

Any changes in symptoms at end of week?

Week Three – Nicotine

Products eliminated Cigarettes, tobacco, passive smoking.

Any changes in symptoms at end of week?

Week Four – Alcohol

Products eliminated Wine, liqueurs, spirits, fortified wines, alcohol products.

Any changes in symptoms at end of week?

Week Five – Caffeine

Products eliminated Coffee, tea, colas, cold relief remedies, cough medicines, any products containing caffeine.

Any changes in symptoms at end of week?

Week Six – Chocolate

Products eliminated Cocoa, chocolate, chocolate biscuits, chocolate drinks, any products containing cocoa/chocolate.

Any changes in symptoms at end of week?

Week Seven – Sugar

Products eliminated Sugar, malt, syrup, treacle, glucose, refined carbohydrates, any products containing sugar.

Any changes in symptoms at end of week?

Week Eight – Colourings and Additives

Products eliminated Highly processed foods, artificially coloured foods, beauty products containing colours.

Any changes in symptoms at end of week?

Week Nine – Stabilisation

Reintroduction Programme

Week One – Dairy

Products reintroduced Milk, butter, cheese, yoghurt, dairy products, low-fat spread, anything containing dairy.

Any changes in symptoms?

Week Two – Grains

Products reintroduced Wheat, flour, bread, corn, corn oil, rye, oats, barley, rice, products containing grains.

Any changes in symptoms?

Week Three – Nicotine

Products reintroduced Cigarettes, tobacco, passive smoking.
Any changes in symptoms?

Week Four – Alcohol

Products reintroduced Wine, liqueurs, spirits, fortified wines, alcohol products.
Any changes in symptoms?

Week Five – Caffeine

Products reintroduced Coffee, tea, colas, cold relief remedies, cough medicines, any products containing caffeine.
Any changes in symptoms?

Week Six – Chocolate

Products reintroduced Cocoa, chocolate, chocolate biscuits, chocolate drinks, any products containing cocoa/chocolate.
Any changes in symptoms?

Week Seven – Sugar

Products reintroduced Sugar, malt, syrup, treacle, glucose, refined carbohydrates, any products containing sugar.
Any changes in symptoms?

Week Eight – Colourings and Additives

Products reintroduced Highly processed foods, artificially coloured foods, beauty products containing colours.

Any changes in symptoms?

WHAT NEXT?

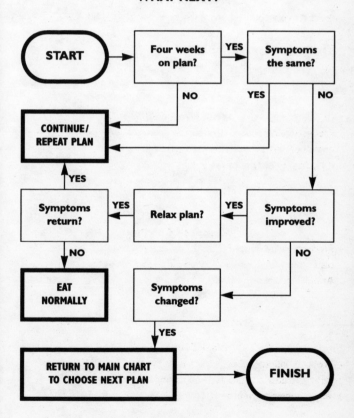

10. The Special Requirements Eating Plan

SPECIAL REQUIREMENTS PLAN CHECK CHART

This chapter deals with those who have special medical or health requirements. Use the check chart below to discover which section is most applicable to your needs. If you have a medical condition which is not mentioned here or elsewhere in the book, and you are not sure if nutrition might affect it, discuss it with your family doctor.

☐   I am a serious competitive athlete. *Go to High Nutrition (p. 280)*

☐   I am diabetic. *Go to Medical Nutrition (p. 284)*

☐   My job is intensive in manual labour. *Go to Eating for Work (p. 286)*

☐   I suffer from kidney stones. *Go to The Calcium Question p. 286)*

☐   I have gout. *Go to Medical Nutrition (p. 284)*

☐   I regularly drink more than three units of alcohol per day. *Go to Alcohol (p. 288)*

☐   I am pregnant. *Go to High Nutrition (p. 280)*

☐   I have been diagnosed HIV positive. *Go to High Nutrition (p. 280)*

☐   I am recovering from serious illness. *Go to High Nutrition (p. 280)*

☐   I have a chronic illness for which I am under regular medical supervision. *Go to Medical Nutrition (p. 284)*

NOTE: Cancer is not included as a nutritionally affected condition in this book. However, there is considerable medical debate at the moment over whether cancer is (a) in part caused by dietary factors, (b) can be alleviated by high (sometimes referred to as super) nutrition. On pp. 334–42 you will find helpful addresses and suggestions for reading reflecting current thinking on cancer.

HIGH NUTRITION

For Athletes

If you honestly are in training (not just the occasional swimming session or weekly aerobics class), you need a healthy diet. But because you are fit, symptoms that you are not eating correctly may be less obvious. For example, many athletes can get away with a diet high in junk food because they metabolise the excess fats and sugars and do not become overfat. But they may still be going short of vital tissue building nutrients.

Athletes should go on a high nutrition diet based on the Low-processing Eating Plan (p. 152) with the addition of the following High Nutrition foods.

High Nutrition Foods

Foodstuff	Vitamin Content	Mineral Content	Nutrition	Other Elements
Carrots	A		Fibre	
Liver	A B1 (thiamine) B2 (riboflavin) Biotin	Zinc	Protein	Lecithin

Foodstuff	Vitamin Content	Mineral Content	Nutrition	Other Elements
Oily fish	A B3 (niacin) B6 (pyridoxine) B12 Biotin D E	Calcium	Protein	Lecithin
Yoghurt	A B2 (riboflavin)	Calcium		Potassium Phosphorus Chloride
Parsley	A C	Iron	Fibre	
Spinach/spring greens	A B2 (riboflavin) Folic acid Bioflavinoids C E		Fibre	
Tomatoes	A Bioflavinoids E			

Foodstuff	Vitamin Content	Mineral Content	Nutrition	Other Elements
Wheatgerm	B1 (thiamine) B2 (riboflavin) B3 (niacin) B6 (pyridoxine) Folic acid Biotin E	Manganese zinc		
Nuts, seeds and pulses	B2 (riboflavin)	Calcium	Protein Fibre Carbohydrate	Potassium
Brown rice	B1 (thiamine) B3 (niacin) B6 (pyridoxine) E		Protein Fibre Carbohydrate	Lecithin Potassium
Bananas	B6 (pyridoxine)	Manganese	Fibre Carbohydrate	Potassium
Oranges	Folic acid Bioflavinoids C		Fibre	
Beans and peas	Folic acid B6 (pyridoxine)	Manganese	Fibre Carbohydrate Protein	

Foodstuff	Vitamin Content	Mineral Content	Nutrition	Other Elements
Green peppers	Bioflavinoids C		Fibre	
Watercress	C		Fibre	

For Pregnancy

Current medical thinking implicates poor nutrition in many pregnancy problems and birth defects. For example, deficiency in B complex vitamins is now linked with spina bifida. Some researchers also believe that nutrition in the 3 months before conception can also improve the chances of a healthy pregnancy and a healthy baby.

If you are planning a pregnancy, you may want to consider the same high nutrition diet as athletes (p. 280). You should also give up smoking and drinking 3–6 months before conception. For more information about planned conception, see p. 338.

If you are already pregnant your ante-natal clinic will have advised you on nutrition. Obviously you should give up smoking and drinking. The Low-processing Eating Plan (p. 152) should be suitable for you. In addition you may be advised to take supplements of B complex vitamins and iron.

WARNING: when pregnant do not take any vitamin supplements or alternative health products without consulting your doctor. Excess of vitamin A can be harmful to your baby. Do not use products containing vitamin A. Beauty and skin care products often contain vitamin A, particularly products which include 'retin . . . ' in their name.

If you are already 3–7 months pregnant the most important
phases in your baby's development are either over or yet to come.
Obviously you should maintain your healthy eating and not
smoke, but the occasional glass of wine is usually permitted.

For HIV and Convalescence

The functioning of the immune system is extremely important in
cases of both an HIV positive diagnosis and convalescence from
a serious illness. The aim is for the immune system to work as
efficiently as possible, and in order to achieve this good nutrition
is essential. A diet rich in vitamins, pro-vitamins and trace
elements will help the body to build new cells and repair tissue as
quickly and efficiently as possible.

If you are recovering from a serious illness, talk about
nutrition to your doctor. If he has no specific recommendations,
follow the advice under High Nutrition (p. 280).

If you have been diagnosed HIV positive, you should discuss
diet and lifestyle with your counsellor or doctor or with an
advice organisation. Useful addresses and reading are listed on p.
338. Current medical thinking is that the state of the immune
system plays an important role in whether and when full-blown
AIDS is developed, and keeping the immune system functioning
as well as possible can deter its onset. Some researchers even
believe that having an immune system impaired by nutrition and
lifestyle factors is a risk factor in HIV.

If you think you are at risk of HIV or have been diagnosed
positive, you should certainly follow a High Nutrition diet (see p.
280). You may also need to make lifestyle changes which are not
in the scope of this book. GET ADVICE, AND FOLLOW IT.

MEDICAL NUTRITION

Diabetics have special dietary requirements which should be
discussed with your family doctor. If you are not diabetic but
have a history of it in the family, you should choose the Low-

sugar Eating Plan (p. 97) and have regular medical check-ups. **Gout** is not an out-of-date problem. It is caused by an excess of uric acid in the blood and you should discuss your eating and drinking with your family doctor.

This is not a medical textbook. If you are seriously or chronically ill, see your family doctor. You may find much that is helpful in this book, but it is no substitute for medical advice. However, coming from a medical background I know that doctors and their patients often have difficulty in communicating with each other. Doctors are highly educated. They train for a minimum of six years before qualification, and even after that most doctors continue to train and research, often for the rest of their lives. They are highly skilled, highly trained and highly dedicated, but no one said they had to be public relations experts. Here are some hints for creating a successful relationship with your doctor.

- Be absolutely honest with yourself and your doctor. If you are not honest the diagnosis and the treatment may be wrong and it will be *your* fault.
- Ask yourself whether you are honestly physically ill. Or are you not really physically ill but unhappy all the same? Your doctor can help with both situations, but only if you reveal honestly which is the true problem.
- Try to be specific about what is wrong. Why do you feel bad? What feels worst? The more precise you can be the easier it is for the doctor to diagnose, and the more he will respect you.
- Remember, if you have decided you need to see a doctor you are almost certainly not at your best, so try not to be too hasty in your judgements.
- Listen carefully to what your doctor says and DO WHAT HE SAYS. If you do not understand what he says, ask him

politely to explain it more simply. If he wants you to do something abstract, like trying to avoid stress, think carefully about ways you might do it and try your best to put them into action.

- When your doctor prescribes a medicine, take it how and when it has been prescribed. No medicine can cure you from the bathroom cabinet.

- If your doctor refers you to another expert, such as a specialist consultant or a family therapist, keep the appointment and TAKE THE ADVICE YOU ARE OFFERED.

- If your doctor wants you to have hospital tests, get them done promptly and make sure the testers know where to send the results.

- Respect your doctor and he will respect you.

- Remember who the expert is. Just because you may have read a magazine article about your problem, or even this book, doesn't make you a professional. Like grannies, doctors do not appreciate being taught how to suck eggs. However, I've never yet met a doctor who doesn't love talking about medicine, so if you have any queries from your reading raise them constructively and you will get your doctor's full attention.

EATING FOR WORK

Manual labour and hard work outdoors mean an increased calorie requirement. If you are overfat it is likely to be because you are eating the wrong foods rather than too much. Start with the Low-sugar or Low-fat Eating Plans (pp. 97, 74) for 4 weeks, and aim to end up stabilising on the Low-processing Eating Plan (p. 152).

THE CALCIUM QUESTION

Kidney stones are usually caused by an excess of calcium or oxalic acid in the system. Most sufferers are recommended to go on a diet low in calcium and drink plenty of fluids. Your family doctor will give you a special nutrition sheet.

Calcium-rich Foods to Avoid

Food Group	Food
Carbohydrate group	Bran, bread (not French bread), wheat flour (not rye flour), wheat-based crispbreads and crackers, pastry, muesli, wheat-flour based biscuits
Vegetable group	Spring onions, spinach, lemons, rhubarb, figs, watercress
Protein group	Soya beans, chick peas, Brazil nuts, almonds, haddock, smoked salmon, seafood, pilchards, sardines, egg yolks
Dairy group	Cheese, milk, yoghurt, chocolate, ice-cream, cocoa, chocolate powder
Added fats	None
Condiments	Soy sauce, molasses, treacle

Oxalic foods to avoid

Carbohydrate group	None
Vegetable group	Red cabbage, rhubarb, beetroot, spring onions, tomatoes, strawberries, dried apricots
Protein group	Peanuts, liver, eggs
Dairy group	None
Added fats	None
Condiments	Mayonnaise

ALCOHOL

Try to be as honest as possible with yourself about your drinking.
You may not think it is excessive but have family and friends
commented? Do you regularly have hangovers? Have you
stopped getting hangovers even though your drinking has not
decreased? Is your memory erratic?

Healthy start

Not only is excess of alcohol unhealthy in itself, but it also has
two effects on nutrition which can lead to deficiencies that
aggravate the problems caused by excess alcohol. Regular over-
use of alcohol depletes the body of vitamins and trace elements.
Long-term over-use of alcohol also tends to decrease the appetite
and saps the will to eat healthily.

   If you regularly and heavily use alcohol, whether or not you
think you over-use it, you should pay serious attention to your
eating:

* Eat regularly, whether you feel like it or not. Four times a
  day is best.
* Decide how much you will eat and of what. Prepare it and
  then serve it in single portions.
* Don't leave anything that you have served yourself to eat.
* Don't make extra meals at odd hours.
* Opt for the Low-processing Eating Plan (p. 152), and in
  addition make sure you have plenty of protein.
* Take a recognised multi-vitamin and mineral supplement.
* Force yourself to drink a glass of water before you have
  alcoholic drink.

Be kind to yourself

The first step in any rehabilitation process is to be kind to yourself. Don't blame yourself. Don't lacerate yourself with guilt. Simply accept the real situation at face value. The most important and worthwhile thing you can do for yourself is confront the real truth about your situation. Then you can begin to do something about it. Do you know in your heart of hearts that your drinking is becoming a problem? Make a bargain with yourself. Complete the check chart (overleaf) honestly. But before you know what the answers indicate, promise yourself that you will accept the diagnosis, whatever it may be.

		do not agree	agree	agree strongly
1	I never drink before a certain time of day.	☐	☐	☐
2	I drink every day.	☐	☐	☐
3	I would be worried if I saw my teenage daughter drink occasionally.	☐	☐	☐
4	I try not to make appointments for after lunch.	☐	☐	☐
5	My sleep is often interrupted.	☐	☐	☐
6	Friends sometimes comment on my clumsiness.	☐	☐	☐
7	I don't really notice if I go a few days without a drink.	☐	☐	☐
8	When visitors come round I sometimes forget to have drink on hand for them.	☐	☐	☐
9	Drink affects my mood quite a lot.	☐	☐	☐
10	I know when I've drunk too much because I get a foul hangover.	☐	☐	☐
11	People are sometimes surprised by my habits.	☐	☐	☐
12	My concentration is poor.	☐	☐	☐
13	I often lose track of things.	☐	☐	☐
14	I keep very regular hours.	☐	☐	☐

Now look at the grid to work out whether your answers are mainly As, mainly Bs or mainly Cs.

ANSWER CODE GRID

	Not agree	Agree	Agree strongly
1	A	C	B
2	C	A	B
3	C	A	B
4	C	B	A
5	C	B	A
6	C	A	B
7	A	C	B
8	A	C	B
9	C	A	C
10	A	B	C
11	C	B	A
12	C	B	A
13	C	B	A
14	A	C	B

Interpretation

Mostly As: You don't really need this book to tell you that you have an alcohol over-use problem. What you do need to do is face the fact and keep your promise to try to follow advice. The first thing to do is accept your problem without guilt or self-blame. You have an illness and what you need is treatment, not judgement or moralising. It doesn't matter how you reached this stage, or how angry or guilty you feel about it. What does matter is trying to overcome it. Don't try to do it on your own. Get help. Turn to p. 338 for addresses and phone numbers.

Mostly Bs: You seem to have an ambivalent and perhaps questionable attitude towards alcohol. It may be that someone in your family has over-used alcohol or you are uncertain about whether you can cope with alcohol. Try to be aware of your health and nutrition, and remember that keeping your body fit and well is a great booster of self-esteem.

Mostly Cs: Either you have a perfectly straightforward attitude to alcohol and are unlikely to have any real problems with your drinking, or you have not answered the questions honestly. Do yourself a favour, tell yourself the truth.

WHAT NEXT?

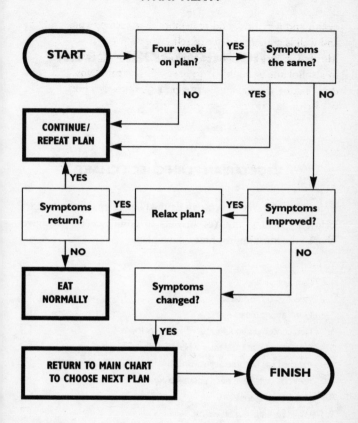

II. The Vegetarian Eating Plan

VEGETARIAN PLAN CHECK CHART

Before you start the Vegetarian Eating Plan, fill in the check chart below by ticking any Yes answers to double-check you have chosen the most appropriate eating plan.

1. I am vegetarian. ☐
2. I want to be vegetarian. ☐
3. I can't afford meat. ☐
4. I am concerned about factory farming methods. ☐
5. I've noticed that I feel fitter when I cut down on meat. ☐
6. My child has become vegetarian. ☐
7. Previous diets have been unsatisfactory. ☐
8. I have fainting spells. ☐
9. I have recently put on weight. ☐
10. I am constantly cold and lethargic. ☐

Ticks KEY

1–3 Unless your Yes answers included 1 and 2, there is probably no particular reason for you to adopt the Vegetarian Eating Plan. However, vegetarian eating is generally healthy. Many people spend 2 or 3 weeks eating vegetarian every year, often after Christmas or in the summer. Why not give it a try?

4–8 The Vegetarian Eating Plan is ideal for you. If you answered Yes to 4, don't forget that humanely farmed meat is now widely available. See Addresses (p. 339).

9–10 If you are already vegetarian and answered Yes to 8 or 10, you may be deficient in certain nutrients. Lack of iron can cause anaemia. Strict vegans will know that they should take vitamin B12 supplement, since this is not naturally available in their diet.

WELCOME TO THE VEGETARIAN EATING PLAN

There are many reasons for going on the Vegetarian Eating Plan, but for me the best reason is how healthy it will make you feel. Although I am not a moral or political vegetarian I regularly go on the Vegetarian Eating Plan for 2 or 3 weeks about three times a year.

Periods of vegetarian eating have tremendous benefits. Your digestion improves, constipation disappears, your skin and hair look healthy. If you return to meat eating afterwards it is with renewed appreciation.

Nutritionists believe that in the West we eat too much meat. Humans do not need meat as a staple source of nutrition in the way that we do carbohydrates and vegetables. Looking at our early ancestors it is likely that meat was a treat food, an exciting extra when it could be obtained, but not something to be relied upon. The reason for this is that meat comes from other living animals. That means that in order to get hold of your meat you must first catch your animal (it may take a dim view of this, and it may even catch you). Then it must be killed and butchered. Meat also takes a long time to digest (especially if it is raw), so you are out of action for some time after eating meat, while you digest (this is why the cat family, pure carnivores, need to be static for around 16 hours a day).

So there are a lot of drawbacks to eating meat, though these are partially outweighed by the fact that meat is such a good source of high-quality protein.

In ecological terms meat is also a very energy-intensive food source. In order to create meat protein an animal must graze on large amounts of protein and carbohydrate provided by grains and grasses. Ecological vegetarians argue that it would be less wasteful and better for the planet if we cut out the middle man, so to speak, and grazed on the grains and grasses ourselves.

Therefore there are very good reasons ecologically and biologically why mankind should naturally be vegetarian. Yet you can tell from our teeth and digestive systems that we are not naturally vegetarian. Our teeth and the size of our stomach and arrangement of our intestines are adapted for an omnivorous diet – that is, we have been used to eating anything and everything we could get our hands on.

The problem today is that man is far less omnivorous than he used to be. Particularly in the West, man has become carnivore biased and eats from a comparatively limited range of foodstuffs. For me, nutritionally speaking, the very best reason for going on the Vegetarian Eating Plan is to restore balance to the diet; to broaden the range of foodstuffs from which we eat and to put meat into its true nutritional perspective.

For many other people, the main reason for trying vegetarianism is moral. I do sympathise with this view. As I write, my two cats are neatly curled up on either side of my desk, and I would never want to inflict pain or suffering on them or any other animal. Yet I have watched these two cuddly cats tease a mouse for half an hour before the creature eventually died of stress. By providing a safe home and additional food for my cats am I condoning and contributing to the suffering they inflict on small mammals? Man's dominant position among the species on this planet causes us endless dilemmas.

Committed vegetarians believe that man has no right to farm animals in any way. But man's interaction with the animal world extends far beyond farming or eating animals. If the non-animal cultivation view is taken to its logical extent, can there be any defence for the keeping of pets?

Further than this, what about man's intervention in the animal world as a whole? Could the breeding operations and conservation projects to save vanishing species be in fact classified as the cultivation of animals? If such projects are not classified as animal cultivation, then the question of the domestication of animals generally has to be looked at again, since some species (including flightless fowl, specialised feeders and pre-historically domesticated animals) would certainly have become extinct without human intervention in the form of farming and domestication.

Like it or not, man is already in a position of guardianship over many species of animal. If the eating of animal products ceased tomorrow, what would happen to all the cows, pigs, chickens and sheep currently being farmed? One committed vegetarian suggested to me in all seriousness that the animals should be turned loose and left to fend for themselves.

As dominant species man interacts with animals in a variety of ways. I think it is our responsibility to behave honourably in all these dealings. It is simply not realistic to think of abandoning farming, but what we can do is ensure that farming is completely free from suffering for the animal involved. That means campaigning for and supporting non-factory farming coupled with humane slaughtering. Please support the following principles:

- No intensive indoor rearing (e.g. veal production).
- No unnatural crowding of animals.
- No artificial suppression of endemic disease, especially where the farming method is conducive to such disease.

- No live mass transportation and export of animals before slaughter.
- No large-scale slaughter houses.
- All deaths to be guaranteed instantaneous.
- Hygienic and respectful handling of carcasses.

By reducing the amount of meat you eat and then by being very careful of the origin of this meat you can make a concrete contribution to these principles. Check out the addresses on pp. 338–9 to find out more about humanely farmed food.

STEP-BY-STEP GUIDE TO THE VEGETARIAN EATING PLAN

1 Read all sections of the diet carefully.
2 Learn what the stop foods are and why you must stop them.
3 Get familiar with all the substitutes and where to buy them.
4 Go through the week-long sample eating programme and work out how it will fit into your lifestyle.
5 If you are at all uncertain you can decide to follow the sample eating programme exactly for a week until you get the hang of things.
6 Learn how to make the snack substitutes.
7 Make a copy of the glance guide to stop and substitute foods.
8 Take the glance guide shopping with you to make sure you are stocking up on the right foods.
9 Remember that any food not mentioned as a stop food can be eaten whenever you like.
10 Note which drinks are to be stopped.
11 Eat plenty of fresh vegetables, these are not stop foods.
12 Follow the diet for as long as you feel comfortable with it, but watch out for symptoms of iron or vitamin deficiency and if you decide to stay on the plan permanently have a regular medical check.

STOP, THINK, SUBSTITUTE

Which foods should I stop eating and what should I substitute?

The Basic Vegetarian Programme

Vegetarians do not eat meat, meat products, meat extracts, meat stocks or animal fats. We all know enough nutrition to know most of the foods that are meat-based. Careful label reading also reveals foods that may surprisingly contain meat. These include tinned soups made with meat stock, cheese made with animal rennet, and some convenience foods that use animal products for thickening and emulsifying.

The basic version of the Vegetarian Eating Plan is fairly easy to follow. Cut out meats and products containing meat and animal fat. Since meat is a major source of protein in the diet, try to make your substitute foods as high as possible in protein. These alternative protein sources include: fish; eggs; vegetarian cheese; rice; nuts; bean sprouts; beans and pulses.

Nutritionists recommend you to use as varied a range of protein sources as possible. Other than that, your eating does not have to change.

NOTE: If you are a committed political vegetarian your lifestyle will also have to be adjusted to preclude the wearing of leather and animal skin products unless you can be certain that the skin is made available as a by-product of the animal's death from natural causes.

- **Stop**: All meats; meat products, animal fats; animal rennet cheese.

- **Substitute**: Fish; eggs; rice; nuts; bean sprouts; beans and pulses; vegetable fats and olive oil; vegetarian cheese.

Non-flesh Vegetarianism

Some vegetarians believe it is wrong to eat the tissue of any animal – flesh, fish or fowl. For that reason they also add fish to the list of foods they do not eat.

- **Stop**: Fish.
- **Substitute**: Non-flesh protein sources.

Non-animal Cultivation Vegetarianism

To cultivate an animal is basically to farm it for food in the way you would a plant. This does not necessarily mean the death of the animal. The animal can be harvested regularly (in the way you would fruit from a tree) to produce a crop which can be wool, hair, milk, eggs, plasma (for medicine), serum (for medicine), sperm (used occasionally as an emulsifier).

Some people believe that it is utterly wrong to cultivate animals in any way. They think that all animals should live in a naturally wild state. Obviously this means they will not eat any animal product at all, including dairy, etc. However, the belief must also have far-reaching effects on lifestyle. Animal products like wool or leather cannot be worn, nor can they be used for any other human purpose.

Not only must the non-animal cultivation vegetarian oppose vivisection, but he must also refuse to be prescribed with any drug that has been developed using vivisection at any stage in the process. Nor logically should he allow himself to be prescribed with any medical vaccine or serum that uses an animal or an animal's blood to develop anti-bodies. Nor indeed should he allow himself to be operated upon by a surgeon whose training has included animal dissection.

- **Stop**: Eggs; dairy products; animal products in medicines.
- **Substitute**: Other sources of protein and calcium; synthetic medicines.

NOTE: A vitamin B12 supplement should also be taken, since this is not available in a diet free from animal products.

AT-A-GLANCE GUIDE TO
STOP AND SUBSTITUTE FOODS

Stop – *Substitute*

Protein Food Group

all meats – *pulses/nuts/beans/bean sprouts*
meat products – *ready-prepared vegetable dishes*
fish (optional) – *pulses/nuts*
eggs (optional) – *as a snack raw vegetables*

Vegetable Food Group

dripping/lard-fried chips – *vegetable-oil-fried chips*

Dairy Food Group

milk/milk products (optional) – *fruit juices*
cheese (optional) – *vegetarian cheese*
dripping/lard – *vegetable oil*
suet – *vegetable oil*

Condiments

Bovril – *Marmite/Vegemite*
stock – *vegetable stock*

NOTES:
- Check labels – some unexpected products contain animal-extracted ingredients. Animal fats and organ extracts are sometimes used as thickening and creaming ingredients in processed food products. If in doubt, leave it out.
- As a vegetarian your sources of protein are more complicated than for meat eaters. You will be relying mainly on a mix of 'second-class' protein sources. As long as you eat a wide variety of these your nutrition will be just as good, if not better, than if you were eating 'first-class' protein. Tips for vegetarian recipes are listed on p. 323.

- WARNING: Many vegetarians find organising their protein sources time-consuming and complicated. They tend to fall back on carbohydrates as filling staples. Make sure you keep a sensible balance of carbohydrate, protein and vegetables in your diet.

SAMPLE SUBSTITUTION PROGRAMME

* Items marked with an asterisk are given in greater detail in the Snack Substitutes and Recipes sections (pp. 313, 324).

MONDAY

Breakfast

Normal 2 slices wholemeal toast with butter and marmalade; cereal with milk; sweetened orange juice; coffee with milk and sugar

Stop (optional) Butter

Substitute Vegetable margarine if desired

Elevenses

Normal 1 biscuit; coffee with milk and sugar

Stop (optional) Butter (in biscuit, check label), milk

Substitute Crispbread with peanut butter

Lunch

Normal Bowl of vegetable soup; sausage roll and salad; apple; 1 glass wine

Stop Sausage roll

Substitute Bowl of soup; large bean sprout salad (with optional cottage cheese); orange; sparkling mineral water

Afternoon tea

Normal Piece of cake; cup of tea without sugar

Stop Milk

Substitute *2 rice cakes spread with honey; cup of tea, lemon

Dinner

Normal Prawn cocktail with 2 slices brown bread; pasta in tomato sauce with courgettes; ice-cream

Stop (optional) Prawns, dairy ice-cream (some ice-creams do not include dairy)

Substitute Avocado vinaigrette with 2 slices brown bread and margarine; *pasta in tomato sauce with courgettes; non-dairy ice-cream sprinkled with unsalted nuts

TUESDAY

Breakfast

Normal 1 soft-boiled egg with 2 slices bread and butter; fresh orange juice; coffee

Stop (optional) Egg

Substitute Porridge; 2 slices toast with margarine; fresh orange juice; coffee

Elevenses

Normal American-style cookie; coffee

Stop (optional) Cookie

Substitute Orange; non-dairy biscuit; coffee

Lunch

Normal Fried chicken limb in breadcrumbs; chips; peas; individual portion fruit trifle; glass wine; coffee

Stop Chicken, animal fat fried chips

Substitute *Mushroom risotto; watercress salad; baked potato (optional cheese topping); peas; trifle (fruit salad if preferred); wine; sparkling mineral water; coffee

Afternoon tea

Normal Small bar of chocolate; tea

Stop (optional) Chocolate

Substitute *Banana and Ryvita sandwich

Dinner

Normal Packet of potato crisps; sausages; baked beans; 2 slices toast; flavoured jelly; 2 glasses wine; coffee

Stop Potato crisps, sausages

Substitute Mixed handfuls of unsalted nuts and olives; *stir-fried barbecue bean curd; baked beans; 2 slices toast; flavoured jelly; 2 glasses wine; coffee

WEDNESDAY

Breakfast

Normal Cereal with milk; pancake with maple syrup; fresh squeezed orange juice; coffee

Stop (optional) Milk, egg

Substitute Cereal with orange juice; 2 grilled potato cakes with maple syrup, banana and nuts; fresh squeezed orange juice; coffee

Elevenses

Normal Shortcake biscuit; coffee

Stop (optional) Shortcake biscuit

Substitute *Rice cake spread with honey; coffee

Lunch

Normal Scotch egg salad; 2 slices brown bread; apple; wine; coffee

Stop Scotch egg

Substitute *Falafel; large continental salad; 2 slices brown bread; apple; mineral water; coffee

Afternoon tea

Normal Snack bar; tea

Stop Check ingredients on label

Dinner

Normal Bowl of vegetable soup; grilled lamb chop; spinach; mashed potato; tinned tomato; fresh unsugared fruit salad; coffee

Stop Lamb chop
Substitute Bowl of vegetable soup; *chilli bean casserole; spinach; mashed potato; tinned tomato; fresh unsugared fruit salad; coffee

THURSDAY

Breakfast

Normal 2 rashers of bacon and 1 fried egg on toast; fresh orange juice; coffee
Stop Bacon (egg)
Substitute *Grilled mushroom cups stuffed with ground hazelnuts and olive oil; egg (or tomato) on toast; fresh orange juice; coffee

Elevenses

Normal Chocolate digestive biscuit; coffee
Stop (optional) Biscuit
Substitute 2 Ryvitas spread with honey (and optional flavoured cottage cheese); coffee

Lunch

Normal Baked potato with cheese; salad; chocolate gâteau; coffee; Coca Cola
Stop (optional) Cheese, chocolate gâteau
Substitute Baked potato with tomato; salad; *mashed banana (with yoghurt) and crumbled oatcake; coffee; Coca Cola

Afternoon tea

Normal Egg sandwich; tea
Stop (optional) Egg
Substitute Salad sandwich; tea

Dinner

Normal Taramasalata with brown bread; commercially prepared cod and salmon fish pie; spinach; grilled tomatoes; ice-cream; 2 glasses wine; coffee; after-dinner mint
Stop (optional) Taramasalata, fish, ice-cream (if dairy), mint (check ingredients)

Substitute Hummus (Greek chick pea spread from supermarkets) with brown bread; *vegetable lasagne; spinach; grilled tomatoes; non-dairy ice-cream; 2 glasses wine; coffee; tangerine

FRIDAY

Breakfast

Normal Toast with jam; coffee
Stop None
Substitute None

Elevenses

Normal Apple; coffee
Stop None
Substitute None

Lunch

Normal Pork pie with chutney; tomato salad; 2 glasses wine; coffee
Stop Pork pie
Substitute Rice salad; tomato salad; 2 glasses wine; coffee

Afternoon tea

Normal Ginger biscuit; tea
Stop (optional) Ginger biscuit
Substitute Ryvita and Marmite/Vegemite; tea

Dinner

Normal 3 measures spirit; Chinese take-away; 2 glasses wine; coffee
Stop Any meat based Chinese dishes
Substitute 3 measures spirit (if you must); Chinese take-away concentrating on stir-fried vegetables; bean curd dishes; vegetable fried rice; vegetable chow mein; vegetable spring roll; vegetable chop suey; 2 glasses wine; coffee

SATURDAY

Breakfast

Normal 1 slice toast; coffee
Stop None
Substitute None

Elevenses

Normal Doughnut; coffee
Stop None
Substitute None

Lunch

Normal Pub lunch of bread, cheese, chutney, salad, chips; ½ pint shandy
Stop Cheese (optional); chips
Substitute Pizza (no cheese); chutney; salad; ½ pint shandy

Afternoon tea

Normal Cake; tea
Stop (optional) Cake
Substitute Honey and banana sandwiches made with soda bread; tea

Dinner

Normal 2 measures spirit; avocado filled with prawns; steak; peas; baked potato; grilled tomatoes and mushrooms; ice-cream; 3 glasses wine
Stop Prawns (optional); steak; ice-cream
Substitute 2 measures spirit (it is Saturday after all); avocado vinaigrette; bean burgers (from supermarkets and health food stores); peas; baked potato; grilled tomatoes and mushrooms; fresh fruit salad; 3 glasses wine

SUNDAY

Breakfast

Normal Bacon; sausage; fried bread; grilled tomatoes; orange juice; coffee
Stop Bacon, sausage, fried bread

Substitute Baked beans; olive oil fried mushrooms; olive oil fried bread; grilled tomatoes; fresh squeezed orange juice; coffee

No elevenses today

Lunch
Normal 2 measures spirit; roast pork; mashed potato; cabbage; peas; gravy; apple pie with cream; coffee
Stop Roast pork, gravy, cream (optional)
Substitute 2 measures spirit; *vegetable bake (see recipe on p. 333); peas; *mixed bean sauce (see recipe on p. 33); apple pie; coffee

Afternoon tea
Normal Biscuit; tea
Stop (optional) Biscuit
Substitute I slice toasted soda bread with honey; tea

Dinner
Normal Spanish omelette; salad; bread; cheese; celery; 2 glasses wine
Stop (optional) Egg, cheese
Substitute Stuffed vine leaves (tinned or fresh from supermarkets and delicatessens); salad; bread; unsalted nuts; celery; 2 glasses wine

WHAT NEXT?

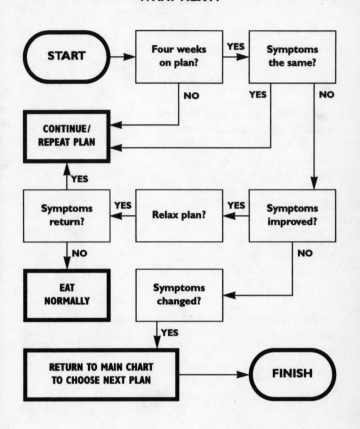

PART THREE

Snack Substitutes

NOTE: those substitutes and recipes containing dairy products would not be suitable for vegans (see p. 300).

For Biscuits

- Savoury *crispbread* (especially brown Ryvita) spread with *honey* and *cottage cheese*. **Suitable for all eating plans.**
- Oat cakes: Patersons sugar-free *oatcakes* from supermarkets. **Suitable for all eating plans.**
- *Crispbreads* spread with diet flavoured low-fat *fromage frais* made by Shape and also own-brand versions – just check to make sure the sweetening is Nutrasweet, not sugar. **NOT suitable for Low-processing Eating Plan.**
- *Rice cakes* spread with diet flavoured low-fat *fromage frais* made by Shape and also own-brand versions, available from the major supermarket chains. **NOT suitable for Low-processing Eating Plan.**
- *Rice cakes* spread with *honey* and *cottage cheese*. **Suitable for all eating plans.**
- *Matzo crackers* spread with *Bovril* (not suitable for vegetarians) and low-fat *cottage cheese*. **Suitable for all eating plans.**

For Cakes / Doughnuts, etc.

- *Granary bread* spread with *honey* and *cottage cheese*. **NOT suitable for Anti-candida Eating Plan.**

- *Fruit*: when you are craving sweet buttery foods like biscuits and cakes, it is well worth trying to acquire a taste for *fruit* instead. Not only is fruit fat-free itself, but there is also some evidence to suggest that the particular kind of soluble fibre it carries is useful in preventing the absorption of fat into the bloodstream. Start off with the less citric fruits – *cherries, peaches*, etc. – eaten with low-fat *yoghurt*. Then try to get yourself to the stage where you can happily snack on *apples* and *oranges*. **Suitable for all eating plans.**

- Chunks of *soda bread* spread with *butter* and *honey*. **NOT suitable for Low-fat Eating Plan or Low-calorie Eating Plan.**

- Continental *bread* spread with lashings of *cream cheese*. **NOT suitable for Low-fat Eating Plan or Low-calorie Eating Plan.**

For Desserts

- A satisfying dessert substitute is plain Greek or similar set *yoghurt* sprinkled with *honey, nuts* and mixed *dried fruit*. **NOT suitable for Low-fat Eating Plan or Low-calorie Eating Plan.**

- Top *fruit salad* and *yoghurts* with home-roasted *nuts, honey* and crumbled *oatcake. Suitable for all eating plans.*

- For an *ice-cream* substitute it is possible to make frozen low-fat yoghurt treats. The simplest way is to take a packet of frozen *raspberries* and, still frozen, whiz them in the blender with a tub of plain low-fat *yoghurt*. If you have a very sweet tooth you can trickle on a little *honey* when you serve. **Suitable for all eating plans.**

- For a crumble substitute, mash *banana* with plain low-fat *yoghurt* and sprinkle with a thick covering of crumbled *oatcake*. **NOT suitable for Menstrual Syndrome Eating Plan.**

- To make *fruit* more satisfying take three different kinds (e.g. *oranges*, *bananas*, peeled sliced *apples*) and stew them together gently in a pan with some *fruit juice*. Serve hot with plain low-fat *yoghurt* and a sprinkling of crumbled *oatcake*. **Suitable for all eating plans.**

- *Frozen yoghurt*: the simplest way to make it is to put a pot of flavoured diet yoghurt in the freezer ready for when you want it. Soften by mashing with a fork before eating. There are some commercially prepared yoghurt ice-creams, but check these for sugar. You can also make yoghurt ice-cream by blending *yoghurt*, *honey* and *fruit purée* and freezing, removing occasionally to beat (use an ice-cream maker if you have one). **NOT suitable for Low-processing Eating Plan.**

- For an ice-cream substitute, take some fresh *fruit* that is naturally sweet. Pulp it and stew it. Pour the pulp into a freezer-proof tub and freeze until it is just soft enough to break up. Turn it into a serving bowl and mash it together with as much *whipped cream/yoghurt/fromage frais* as desired. **NOT suitable for Low-fat Eating Plan or Low-calorie Eating Plan.**

- Any low-sugar pudding can be made more cheerful by topping with *crème chantilly* – this is *cream* which has been whipped together with a generous sprinkling of *vanilla essence*. You could make other flavoured crèmes using *liqueurs*, *peppermint essence*, *Camp coffee essence*, etc. **NOT suitable for Low-fat Eating Plan or Low-calorie Eating Plan.**

For Breakfast Cereals

- *Oat bran flakes*: a couple of years ago there was a great deal of publicity about the value of oats and oat bran in reducing cholesterol levels. The American researchers conjectured that the high levels of soluble fibre available in oats had a tendency to inhibit cholesterol-promoting LDL (low density lipid) fats from being absorbed into the bloodstream. Further research has since suggested that any alteration in diet away from fat and calorie-rich foods to low nutritional density 'third world' foods may achieve the same effect. Whatever the outcome of the debate, the good effect for those on a low-cholesterol diet is that many more oat-based foods are now available in supermarkets. It makes sense to switch to these products. Try to avoid those containing sugar, check diabetic and health food ranges. **Suitable for all eating plans.**

- *Flaked oats* or *rye*: available from health stores and makes a good substitute for muesli mixed with *nuts* and chopped fresh *fruit*. **Suitable for all eating plans.**
- *Puffed wheat*: sugar-free version available from health stores. **NOT suitable for Anti-candida Eating Plan.**
- *Shredded wheat* – the best of all the commercial cereals. **NOT suitable for Anti-candida Eating Plan.**
- Any unsweetened *muesli*. *Suitable for all eating plans.*

For Chocolate

- *Cheese*. **NOT suitable for Low-fat Eating Plan.**
- *Banana*. **NOT suitable for Menstrual Syndrome Eating Plan.**
- *Banana sandwich*: Pulp your *banana* and sandwich between two slices of *brown bread*. **NOT suitable for Menstrual Syndrome Eating Plan or Anti-candida Eating Plan.**
- *Banana and Ryvita sandwich*: Pulp your *banana* and sandwich between two slices of brown *Ryvita* crispbread. **NOT suitable for Menstrual Syndrome Eating Plan.**
- *Pineapple rings* with *cream cheese*. **NOT suitable for Low-fat Eating Plan, Low-cholesterol Eating Plan or Low-calorie Eating Plan.**

- Flavoured low-fat diet *yoghurt* sweetened with *Nutrasweet*, not sugar, by Shape or own-brand from major supermarket chains. **NOT suitable for Low-processing Eating Plan.**
- Quartered *orange* with skin on to suck. **Suitable for all eating plans.**
- Sugar-free *chewing-gum*. **NOT suitable for Low-processing Eating Plan.**
- Burnt *toast* spread with runny *honey*. **NOT suitable for Anti-candida Eating Plan.**

For Sandwiches

- *Potato crisps*. **NOT suitable for Low-fat Eating Plan, Low-calorie Eating Plan, Low-cholesterol Eating Plan or Low-processing Eating Plan.**
- *Soda bread sandwiches* – either hunks of *soda bread* stuffed with *salad* or *tuna*, or sandwiches made in the normal way with sliced *soda bread*. **Suitable for all eating plans.**
- Open *crispbread sandwiches* with topping of your choice. **Suitable for all eating plans.**

For Meat Snacks

- *Pepperonis* – continental pure meat sausages instead of British bangers and sausage rolls. **NOT suitable for Low-processing Eating Plan or Vegetarian Eating Plan.**
- *Hamburgers* of pure meat served on *soda bread*, not bread roll. **NOT suitable for Vegetarian Eating Plan, Low-fat Eating Plan, Low-cholesterol Eating Plan or Low-processing Eating Plan.**

For Salad Dressings/Sauces

- Look out for the diet versions of your normal *mayonnaise*, *ketchup* and *salad cream*. Even more low-cal is to make your own dressings and sauces from combinations of the following ingredients: *vinegar, soy sauce, Worcester sauce, lemon juice, orange juice, low-fat yoghurt, mustard, olive oil, thin tomato purée* or *tomato juice*. Experiment with different combinations to go with different dishes. Serve cold over salads and hot over meats and pastas. Don't use too much olive oil. **Suitable for all eating plans.**

For Tomato Purée

- Thin tomato purée is an excellent low-fat substitute for fatty gravies, sauces and stocks. Simplest of all is to buy tins of chopped *tomatoes* and use liberally. You can make your own from skinned fresh tomatoes whizzed in the blender and you can add *parsley, garlic, herbs* and *lemon juice* to taste and keep it fresh in the fridge. **Suitable for all eating plans.**

For Chutney

- Savoury yoghurt dip made by chopping any combination of *herbs, garlic* and *tomato purée* into plain *yoghurt* to taste. **Suitable for all eating plans.**

For Butter

- *Vegetable-oil based spreads* and *margarines* are now widely available. Choose one marked 'high in polyunsaturates' and read the label to make sure the claim is justified. **NOT suitable for Low-processing Eating Plan.**

For Salt

- The first thing to do is check, check, check the label of every food or ingredient that you buy. It isn't just foods that taste salty that include *salt*. Many breakfast cereals, for example, contain hidden salt. Don't buy food that contains salt. Don't add salt either in cooking or at the table. If you must, use a 'low-salt' seasoning available at supermarkets.

Better still, try herbs and spices with your food instead. **Suitable for all eating plans.**

For Peanuts and Junk Snacks

- *Potato crisps* are not especially healthy, but a small pack is only about 120 calories, much less than a packet of peanuts, and therefore a sensible compromise. In general potato crisps are the lesser of two evils when it comes to alternatives like biscuits, chocolate bars and other snack foods. **Suitable for all eating plans.**

For Potato Crisps

- Make sure you always have a bowl of raw *vegetable sticks* (*carrot, celery, bell pepper, sugar peas,* etc.) ready in the fridge to browse on in case of a snack attack. Season with *herbs, barbecue spice* or *black pepper.* Many supermarkets stock these ready prepared and packed, so they are just as convenient as crisps. **Suitable for all eating plans.**
- In bars and pubs, *olives* and *cocktail pickles* are usually available in addition to the normal crisps and peanuts. Leave the crisps and peanuts alone and eat the olives and pickles instead. **Suitable for all eating plans.**
- Nuts: *almonds* and *walnuts,* unroasted or home-roasted if preferred (to roast your own nuts put a dab of *olive* or *sesame oil* in a non-stick frying pan and fry the nuts until they reach a golden-brown; cool a little and sprinkle with *herbs* or *salt*). **NOT suitable for Low-cholesterol Eating Plan.**
- Handfuls of fresh unsalted *olives.* **Suitable for all eating plans.**

For Chips

- Can there ever be a totally satisfying substitute for *chips*? Of course not. But there are some compromises. When eating out, *baked, boiled* and *mashed potatoes* are obvious alternatives. When eating at home you can have *roast stick vegetables* which, while not chips, aren't bad. Take some *carrots* and *parsnips*, cut into sticks and briefly parboil. Put them into an oven dish and brush them with *olive, sesame* or *walnut oil*. Roast in a hot oven until crisp, turning occasionally and brushing on a little extra oil. **Suitable for all eating plans.**

For Scrambled Whole Eggs

- The debate about whether the (dietary) cholesterol in egg yolks contributes to the cholesterol in our blood stream has yet to be fully resolved. For the time being the sensible course seems to be to limit your intake of eggs if you are a big egg-eater. If you only eat eggs once in a while I wouldn't worry about it. You can make scrambled eggs without using the egg yolks (use those for feeding the birds if no one else in your family will have them). Beat up *egg white* with a little *skimmed milk* and *tomato sauce* for colouring. Sprinkle with chopped *herbs*, e.g. *parsley* and then scramble in the normal way in *olive oil*. **Suitable for all eating plans.**

For Hot/Cold Malted/Chocolate Drinks

- Hot *'bouillon'* – thin stock drink either bought as powder from the stocks and gravy section of your supermarket or health store (**NOT suitable for Low-processing Eating Plan**) or made yourself by stewing any combination of vegetables and meat (*see vegetarian notes on p. 323*) and straining off the liquid. Commercial ones tend to be high in salt, so it's best to make your own; it will keep well in the fridge.
- Warm *skimmed milk* flavoured with a couple of drops of *vanilla essence*.

- *Cup soup*, especially low-calorie instant soup mixes. **NOT suitable for Low-processing Eating Plan.**
- *Yoghurt shake* made with plain *yoghurt*, 2 *ice cubes* and any *fruit juice* or *fruit*, blended in a liquidiser. **Suitable for all eating plans.**
- *Milk shake* made with *skimmed milk* and *fruit purée* whizzed together in a blender. **Suitable for all eating plans.**

For Tea and Coffee

There are several *coffee* substitutes on the market, usually made with things like acorns and chicory. If you talk to someone who lived during the war when coffee was difficult to get, they will tell you that what they had instead – 'ersatz' – was foul. They will also tell you it was made with things like acorns and chicory. Having tried the current coffee substitutes I can sympathise with their point of view. As a former coffee addict I have come to the conclusion that it is ultimately more successful to break yourself of the habit altogether. I therefore recommend the following substitutes:

- *Hot lemon* and *honey* made by pouring boiling *water* on to a teaspoon of Jif *lemon juice* and a teaspoon of *honey*.
- *Hot spiced orange* made by pouring ½ glass of boiling *water* on to ½ a glass of pure *orange juice* and sprinkling with *cinnamon* or *mixed spices*.
- *Hot vegetable 'bouillon'* – thin stock drink made by stewing any combination of vegetables and/or meat and straining off the liquid.
- Hot juice drinks made with any combination of *fruit juices* mixed half and half with *hot water*.
- *Tea* is a different matter, since the various *fruit* and *herb teas* now on the market seem very palatable. But I am not a big tea drinker, so my opinion may be suspect.

For Alcohol

- Instead of *wine* or *beer* choose from the following: *diet soft drinks*; *mineral water*; *Piermont* (a sparkling spring water with apple and blackcurrant available at most supermarkets, off-licences and health stores). **NOT suitable for Low-processing Eating Plan.**
- Instead of spirits, choose from the following: *Virgin Mary* (seasoned tomato juice); *pineapple juice*; *orange juice*; any non-alcoholic cocktails (most bars now offer these). **Suitable for all eating plans.**

For Colas and Fizzy Drinks

- Sparkling *fruit juice* and *mineral water*.
- Plain or flavoured *mineral water*.
- Sparkling *mineral water*; pure *orange juice* diluted with *soda water*; diet *tonic water*; *tomato juice*; fruit-flavoured *mineral waters* (check no sugar).

For Tinned Vegetables and Pulses

- Make your own version of tinned *baked beans* by soaking a selection of *dried beans* (*chick peas, black-eyed beans, kidney beans*) overnight, then rinsing and boiling them fiercely until thoroughly softened. Make a sauce of *fried onion, tomato purée, tomato juice* and *lemon juice* thickened with a little *cornflour*, and pour over the beans. **Suitable for all eating plans.**
- *Mixed bean salad* is available from supermarkets in tins or from the chill counter. Check the ingredient list to make sure the sugar is not too high, and use as a quick substitute when you are busy.
- There are also versions of *baked beans* which contain no sugar – check the label.

Additional Notes for Vegetarians

If you are becoming vegetarian only in so far as you are cutting out meat, most of these substitutes will not be relevant, but some vegetarians do not eat any animal products at all, including butter, milk, eggs, dairy chocolate and cheese.

For Butter

- Vegetable-oil based spreads and margarines are now widely available, as are vegetarian cheeses.

For Butter Biscuits and Dairy Cakes

- Rice cakes spread with honey, Marmite or Vegemite.

For Hot and Cold Malted/Chocolate Drinks and Shakes

- Hot vegetable 'bouillon' – thin stock drink either bought as powder or made yourself by stewing any combination of vegetables and straining off the liquid.
- Cup soup, especially low-calorie instant soup mixes.

Recipes

Tzatsiki

Tzatsiki is a Greek dip made mainly with yoghurt. You can either buy it at your supermarket (look for it alongside the taramasalata) or make your own. Recipes vary. My favourite is low-fat *yoghurt* whizzed in the blender with *cucumber, lemon juice* and a couple of sprigs of *fresh mint*.

Low-fat Pork Casserole

Take *fillet pork* and trim off any visible excess fat. Dice into small cubes. Heat 1 tblsp *olive, walnut* or *sesame oil* in a non-stick frying pan. Stir-fry the pork until brown and transfer to an oven-proof casserole. Into the frying pan juices add a selection of diced *vegetables* of your choice (start by trying *onions, cucumber* and *mushrooms*) are stir-fry until soft. Add the vegetables to the casserole. Pour *water, tomato purée* and *herbs* into the frying pan and stir all together until the juices have amalgamated. Pour these pan juices into casserole and top up with *water* or *stock* if you feel it necessary. Cook in a medium oven for about 45 minutes.

Before serving allow to cool a little and stir in a generous dollop of low-fat *yoghurt*. This basic recipe can be adapted to most meats and forms the basis for a low-fat style of cooking.

Home-made Chinese Food

Correctly cooked Chinese food is not as fattening as you might imagine. Think about it – how many of the waiters and waitresses who serve you at Chinese restaurants are overweight? Quite.

If you're not cooking it yourself, choose the following dishes:

- Plain boiled rice, not fried (the Chinese never eat fried rice themselves, so you'll win brownie points with the waiter!).
- Bean curd dishes.
- Stir-fry vegetable dishes.
- Steamed or boiled dishes.

When cooking at home, the basis of any Chinese meal is the quick stir-fry which can be adapted to produce all sorts of different dishes according to ingredients and seasonings. Here is a base recipe on which you can ring the changes.

Heat 1 tablespoon of *sesame oil* in a deep non-stick frying pan. Add a diced *onion* and soften. Then add matchstick-thin strips of lean *beef* and fry until nearly brown. Add diced *tomato* and sliced *green* and *red pepper*. While stir-frying all together, add *soy sauce, sherry, orange juice* and *barbecue sauce* (or *plum, hoisin* or *black bean sauce* if your local supermarket's ethnic section has it). Fry for a few moments until the liquid is more or less gone and the beef is beginning to be well done. Remove from the heat and serve over bowls of boiled *rice*. As you can imagine, this recipe has almost limitless variations.

Cheesecake

Take a flan dish and line the base with a layer of crumbled *oat biscuit*. Chill in the fridge. Meanwhile mix together a tub of *cottage cheese*, plenty of *lemon juice*, some *grated lemon zest* and *honey* to taste. Take a packet of *gelatine* and make it up according to instructions (usually by heating in water). When the gelatine is ready, blend it quickly into the cottage cheese mixture, ensuring there are no lumps. Pour the gelatine and cottage cheese mixture over the oat biscuit base and leave to set. It will not be as sweet as you are used to.

Tomato and Herb Risotto

This is a soft, Italian-style risotto. Use half and half *brown* and *white rice*. Pour the desired amount into a pan of boiling water and boil for 5 minutes. Drain and rinse. In a deep frying pan heat 2 tablespoons *olive oil* (the best you can afford). Sprinkle on any mixture of *dried herbs* you like up to a quantity of about 2 teaspoons. Add *garlic* (chopped or purée from a tube) to taste. Stir-fry briefly. Add the *rice* and stir-fry briefly. Now pour on enough chopped *Italian tomatoes* (available in tins) to cover. Put a lid on the pan and simmer long and gently until the rice has absorbed most of the juice. Stir occasionally to prevent sticking. Meanwhile chop 2 large hard *tomatoes* (preferably green) and a selection of *fresh herbs* (supermarkets usually have a good range available). Stir these into the risotto and serve immediately.

Vegetable Risotto

This is a dry risotto. Use a mixture of *brown, white* and *wild rice* according to your taste (and pocket!). Put the rice into a pan of cold water and bring to boil. Simmer until the grains are just beginning to swell. Drain and rinse. In a frying pan heat a tablespoon of *walnut oil*. Sauté a chopped *onion*. Add 3 medium *carrots*, cut into matchsticks. Keep stirring. Add some *peas* (preferably leftovers). When the vegetables are softening add the rice. It is important to keep stirring so that things don't stick. Pour on enough stock to prevent this. Add chopped *green pepper* and *watercress*. Stir until watercress has wilted and serve.

Fish Pie

Boil and mash some *potatoes* and put to one side. Gently poach any choice of *fish* in a little *skimmed milk* and *stock*. In a separate pan fry a chopped *onion* in a little *olive oil* with *herbs* to taste.

Chop some *cucumber*. Take an ovenproof dish and put a layer of chopped *onion* in the bottom. Then put in alternate layers of the poached *fish* (whole or flaked), the chopped *cucumber* and any remaining *onion* until you are three-quarters of the way up the dish. Take the *juices* from the fish poaching and add *herbs, white wine* and *lemon juice*. Simmer to reduce the juice slightly. Pour over the mixture in the dish and top with *mashed potato*. Lightly brush the potato with *olive oil* and heat through in a hot oven. Do not overcook.

Almond Orange

For a breakfast dish, take the largest *orange* you can find, halve, and prepare as you would a grapefruit. Arrange the two halves on a grillproof tray. Spread thinly with *marmalade* and sprinkle with chopped *almonds*. Put under a high grill for a few moments until the *marmalade* is bubbling and beginning to burn. Serve with low-fat *yoghurt* if desired. You can do the same with grapefruit too.

Mushroom Vinaigrette

If preparing at home, take large *open cup mushrooms*. Remove the stalks and chop them very finely. Stir them into a *vinaigrette sauce* and pour into the mushroom cups. Sprinkle with chopped *parsley*. If in a restaurant, simply ask for a chopped raw mushroom salad with a vinaigrette dressing. **NOT suitable for Anti-candida Eating Plan.**

Chicken and Cucumber Casserole

Skin and finely chop as many *chicken breasts* as you need. Dredge in a little *cornflour*. Heat 1 tablespoon of *sesame oil* in a deep pan. Stir-fry 1 *chopped onion*, some *chopped parsley* and some *chopped green pepper*. Add the *chicken* and stir-fry until browned. Add a *whole sliced cucumber* and continue to stir-fry while the cucumber wilts. Sprinkle with *lemon juice* and *sesame* seeds. Pour on enough *light stock* to cover, and leave to simmer slowly for about 20 minutes. Add only enough extra liquid if necessary to prevent sticking. Pour on $^1/_2$ *a glass of wine* and continue to simmer gently for a couple of minutes. At the last minute stir in a little *low-fat yoghurt* and serve with a garnish of *toasted almonds*. NOT suitable for Vegetarian Eating Plan.

Vegetable Ratatouille

This staple of student life is so simple to prepare that it almost doesn't have a recipe. Just get a selection of *seasonal vegetables* (including salad vegetables if you want) and chop them up into manageable slices. Heat some *oil* in a pan (ring the changes with *walnut, sesame* and *olive oils*). Toss in some *herbs* and *garlic* and then start stir-frying your vegetables. Put in first the ones that take longest to cook (e.g. root vegetables like carrots) and add the quickest cooking ones (like lettuce) last. When all the vegetables are in and the hardest ones are beginning to soften pour on some liquid – it can be whatever you want: *stock, tomato purée, wine, cider, lemon juice* or a mixture – put on the lid and simmer gently until the hardest vegetables are very nearly completely soft. The Italians call this 'al dente'. Don't let it simmer too long or the whole thing will turn into a sludge. Serve it with *warm bread* and a sprinkling of *black pepper*.

Beef Casserole

Take the best cut of *beef* you can afford. Trim off any visible fat. Heat a tablespoon of *olive* or *walnut oil* in a frying pan. Cut the beef into cubes and brown in the hot oil along with your favourite herbs. Remove the meat and place in an ovenproof casserole. Add your choice of *vegetables* to the juices in the frying pan and stir-fry them gently, adding *tomato purée, lemon juice* and a little *water* to prevent burning. When the vegetables are softened, add them to the casserole. Pour some water on to the remaining pan juices and add a variety of *seasonings*. Boil up to

reduce, then pour over the meat and vegetables in the casserole.
Add more liquid if necessary. Cook in a medium oven for about
45 minutes. Ten minutes before the end of cooking, pour off a
little liquid. Allow it to cool and blend in *2 teaspoons cornflour*
before returning it to the pot and finishing cooking. Following
this basic procedure you can use a huge variety of ingredients to
create a range of tasty low-fat dishes. **NOT suitable for
Vegetarian Eating Plan.**

Tuna Salad

Commercially prepared tuna salads in a variety of mixes are
available both tinned and fresh from your supermarket delicatessen counter. They are not especially low-calorie, but on the
whole the fat they contain is olive oil which is not a major
problem. However if you want to be strict you can make your
own tuna salad using *tuna tinned in brine* which you have rinsed
and drained before mixing with your favourite *salad ingredients*
and dressing with your own home-made *low-fat dressing* (see
p.317).

Seafood Salad

Generally you should avoid prawn cocktail as the dressing may
be quite high in fat. Instead opt for plain seafood salad of
prawns, mussels, etc. dressed with *lemon juice* and *black pepper*.

Pasta in Tomato Sauce

Boil some *pasta* in *water* laced with *olive oil*. Drain while still 'al
dente' (not too soft). Put in a dish and stir in more *olive oil* and
fresh herbs. Pour over *tomato purée* made as below. Serve. **NOT
suitable for Anti-candida Eating Plan.**

The Basic Tomato Purée

I have found that on the Low-processing Eating Plan the biggest thing you miss is the convenience of having a wide range of pre-prepared sauces, soups, gravies and flavourings to add to your cooking. At first it is also hard to reproduce the sort of tasty sauces that come with ready-made meals. To combat this I have developed a basic tomato purée which can be made up in batches and kept in the fridge or freezer. It is primarily a sauce but can be used as a cooking liquid, stock, soup base, gravy base or anything that needs a tasty liquid. Here is how to make it.

Skin *1 lb of tomatoes*. Heat *1 teaspoon of olive oil* in a deep pan and stir-fry *mixed herbs* and *chopped parsley*. Add the *tomatoes* and continue to stir-fry. Add a little *lemon juice*. Allow to cool and then whizz to a purée in the blender.

VARIATIONS: Use *mushrooms, cucumbers, aubergines* or *avocados* instead of or as well as tomato.

ADDITIONS: Melt in grated *cheese*; thicken with *milk* and *cornflour*; stir in thick *yoghurt*; add *garlic* or other *seasonings*.

Spare Ribs

Use outdoor-reared *pork spare rib* or *belly* (see p. 336 for addresses). Chop into small riblets, taking care to remove any splinters of bone. Add *honey, orange juice, sherry* to the basic *tomato purée* and marinade overnight in an ovenproof dish. When preparing your meal, take the dish of marinated ribs and roast in a medium oven for 20 minutes. Transfer the ribs to a grill rack and grill fiercely on both sides until the outside is beginning to burn. Excess marinade can be used as a baste or reduced by simmering to pour over finished ribs as a sauce. **NOT suitable for Vegetarian Eating Plan.**

Stuffed Mushrooms

Take large open cup *mushrooms*. Remove and chop up the stalks. Fry the chopped stalks in a generous quantity of *butter* and chopped *parsley*. Pour into the mushroom cups and heat in a medium oven for about 10 minutes. Serve. **NOT suitable for Anti-candida or Low-fat Eating Plans.**

Beansprout Salad

Either sprout your own seeds (packets from garden centres and health stores) or buy beansprouts at your supermarket. Toss into a salad with *cucumber* and *mushroom* chunks and shredded fresh *spinach*. Dress with *lemon juice, soy sauce* and *tomato purée*.

Mushroom Risotto

Parboil, rinse and cool some *rice*. Stir-fry chopped *onion*, whole button *mushrooms* and fresh *parsley*. Add the *rice* and continue to fry together, gradually adding *vegetable stock, garlic purée* and *mushroom purée* until the desired consistency is achieved. If desired you can stir in an *egg*. **NOT suitable for Anti-candida Eating Plan.**

Watercress Salad

Slice an *orange* and toss with torn bunches of *watercress*. Sprinkle with chopped *nuts* and *sesame seeds*. Dress with *sesame oil* and *wine vinegar*.

Stir-fried Barbecue Beancurd

Buy packet of *beancurd* (also labelled tofu) from your super-market, or buy fresh beancurd from a Chinese store if you have one near. Drain and slice. Stir-fry an *onion* and add the *beancurd*. Turn gently to avoid breaking it while you pour on *barbecue sauce*. Serve with *rice* and *vegetables*.

Falafel

Most supermarkets and delicatessen counters now stock this Middle Eastern dish. If you can't get hold of them, try this simple version. Rinse and drain ½ a tin of *broad beans* and ½ a tin of *chick peas* and whiz them in the blender with a chopped *onion*. Add *garlic, parsley, salt, coriander* and *cumin seeds* and whiz again. You should now have a thick chunky paste. If it is too runny add some more chick peas. Take walnut-size nuggets of paste and form into small patties. Fry the patties in *sesame oil* until golden. Serve with *salad*.

Chilli Bean Casserole

Take a tin of *mixed beans* and a tin of *red kidney beans*. Rinse and drain. Fry 2 chopped *onions*. Add the *beans* and some *herbs*. Add whole large *mushrooms* and continue to fry. Add enough *vegetable stock* to cover partially. Now add *chilli sauce* and, if you can get them, whole fresh *green chillis*. Turn the heat down and simmer gently for about 15 minutes. Thicken with *cornflour* if desired.

Grilled Mushroom Cups

Take large open-cup *mushrooms* and paint the inside with *olive oil*. Sprinkle with anything you like – chopped *garlic*, chopped *hazelnuts, parsley* (grated *cheese* if you like), and grill briefly. **NOT suitable for Anti-candida Eating Plan.**

Vegetable Lasagne

Stir-fry sliced *onion, cucumber, tomato* and *mushroom* (and *aubergines* if desired). Parboil *lasagne* strips (they should not be too soft) in water laced with *olive oil* (this will prevent sticking). In an ovenproof dish layer lasagne and vegetable mix, seasoning each layer to taste. Top with raw sliced *tomatoes* (and *cheese* if desired). Cook in a medium oven for about 15 minutes. **NOT suitable for Anti-candida Eating Plan.**

Vegetable Bake

Line an ovenproof dish with a layer of thin-sliced *potato*. Brush with *olive oil*. Then put in alternative layers of fried *onions*, fried *mushrooms*, sliced *tomatoes*. Put your favourite *herbs* in between layers (and *cheese* if desired). Finish with a final layer of sliced *potato*. Brush with *olive oil* and sprinkle with *black pepper*. Bake gently until the potatoes are soft.

Mixed Bean Sauce

Make your own version of tinned baked beans. Take a selection of dried *beans (chick peas, black-eyed beans, kidney beans)*, soak overnight, rinse and boil fiercely until thoroughly softened. Then make a sauce of fried *onion, tomato purée, tomato juice* and *lemon juice* thickened with a little *cornflour* and pour over the beans.

Addresses

1. Low-calorie Eating Plan/Congenital Obesity

MIND
National Association for Mental Health, Granta House, 15–19
Broadway, Stratford, London E15 4BQ. 081 519 2122.
*Dedicated to promoting understanding of those with mental
health difficulties and to providing help for sufferers.*

The British Association of Counsellors Service
1 Regent Place, Rugby CV21 2PJ. 0788 578328.
*Counsellors do not have formal psychiatric qualifications, but
those belonging to the Association will have had training. If your
family doctor is unhelpful, the Association can help with getting
in touch with a reputable counsellor to help with eating
problems, emotional difficulties.*

2. Low-fat Eating Plan

NACNE
c/o Health Education Authority
*Governmental group concerned with the national diet and
health.*

British Dietetic Association
7th Floor, Elizabeth House, 22 Suffolk Street, Queensway, Birmingham B1 1LS. 021 643 5483.
Important body for trained dieticians and can help put individuals in touch with specialist dietary advice.

British Nutrition Foundation
High Holborn House, 52–54 High Holborn, London WC1V 6RQ. 071 404 6504.
Dedicated to furthering research into nutrition and promoting knowledge of healthy eating.

3. Low-sugar Eating Plan/Eating Disorders

Eating Disorders Association
Sackville Place, 44 Magdalen Street, Norwich, Norfolk. 0603 621414.
Set up to provide support and information for those suffering anorexia, bulimia and compulsive eating.

Women's Therapy Centre
6 Manor Gardens, London N7. 071 263 6200.
Takes a woman-centred approach to emotional/health problems, especially eating problems.

Professor Herbert Lacey
Bulimia Clinic
St George's Hospital, London.
One of the foremost authorities on bulimia, and extremely busy, but the clinic does its best to help with information, etc. and your family practitioner might get you a referral.

4. Low-cholesterol Eating Plan

British Heart Foundation
14 Fitzhardinge Street, London W1H 4DH. 071 935 0185.

Main body for the promotion of knowledge on heart/arterial disease and research into how diet is related to the disease. A mine of information.

5. Low-processing Eating Plan

British Society for Allergy and Environmental Medicine
(incorporating the Society for Nutritional Medicine)
Acorns, Romsey Road, Cadnam, Southampton SO40 2NN.
Established in response to findings in the last couple of decades about how poor-quality food and pollutants/contaminants can affect health. Mainly concerned with the exchange of information between professionals, but will help with local contacts, etc.

The Soil Association
86–88 Colston Street, Bristol BS1 5BB. 0272 290661.
The central body concerned with organic farming and food production. Can help with all sorts of information about where to buy organic products and non-factory farmed foods.

Macbeths
Traditional Meat, 20 High Street, Forres, Moray, IV36 0DB. 0309 672254.
A mail order source of good quality meats.

6. Menstrual Syndrome Eating Plan

Elizabeth Garratt Anderson Hospital
PMS Clinic
Dept of Gynaecology, Euston Road, London NW1. 071 387 2501.
A centre of research into PMS and may be able to help with local referrals if London is too far away for you.

Women's Nutritional Advisory Service
PO Box 268, Lewes, East Sussex BN7 2QN. 0273 487366.
*Excellent source of information on eating for health generally,
and closely concerned in finding answers to PMS.*

7. Oral Contraceptive Syndrome Eating Plan

Family Planning Association
27–35 Mortimer Street, London WC1M 7RJ. 071 636 7866.
*General source of contacts and detailed information on oral
contraception.*

8. Anti-candida Eating Plan

G & G Supplies
175 London Road, East Grinstead, West Sussex RH19 1YY.
*Mail order supplier of lactobacillus acidopholus (useful in the
treatment of candida) and other supplements.*

9. Low-allergen Eating Plan

National Eczema Society
5–7 Tavistock Place, London WC1H 9SR. 071 388 4097.
Help and information for eczema sufferers.

National Asthma Campaign
Providence House, Providence Place, London N1 0NT. 071 226
2260.
Research, etc. into asthma and related health problems.

Action Against Allergy
24–26 High Street, Hampton Hill, Middlesex TW12 1PD.
*Involved with the wider spectrum of allergy in addition to those
already recognised by conventional medicine.*

Migraine Trust
45 Great Ormond Street, London WC1 3HD. 071 278 2676.
Support and information for migraine sufferers.

10. Special Requirements Eating Plan

Foresight
Association for Preconceptual Care
28 The Paddock, Godalming, Surrey GU7 1XJ. 048342 7839.
Pioneering voluntary group promoting the theory (now widely accepted) that health and nutritional status at around the time of conception and during pregnancy affects the outcome of the pregnancy. Will do dietary analysis, etc., and provides a great deal of information.

Action on Smoking and Health
109 Gloucester Place, London W1H 3PH. 071 935 3519.
Campaigns against smoking and to encourage people to give up smoking.

The Terrence Higgins Trust
52–54 Grays Inn Road, London WC1X 8JU. 071 831 0330.
The leading AIDS foundation.

Alcohol Concern
275 Grays Inn Road, London WC1X 8QF. 071 833 3471.
Support and information for alcoholics and the families of alcoholics.

11. Vegetarian Eating Plan

The Vegetarian Society
Parkdale, Dunham Road, Altrincham, Cheshire. 061 928 0793.
Central group for the promotion of vegetarianism.

The Soil Association and British Organic Farmers
86 Colston Street, Bristol BS1 5BB. 0272 2906661.
Source of information and contacts for natural farmed foods and vegetarian foods.

Free Range Egg Association
37 Tanza Road, London NW3 2UA. 071 435 2596.
The central body for producers of free range eggs.

12. General Addresses

Health Education Authority
Hamilton House, Mabledon Place, London WC1H 9TX. 071 413 1970.
Key body concerned with the promotion of nutrition and health in this country.

Family Doctor Publications
BMA House, Tavistock Square, London WC1H 9JP. 071 387 9721.
Produces books on specific health issues and will help with queries where possible.

British Holistic Medical Association
179 Gloucester Place, London NW1 6DX. 071 262 5299.
Concerned to promote complementary medicine. If some of the ideas in this book appeal to you particularly, you may find it interesting to study holistic and complementary treatments.

Bibliography

Books

Bender, Arnold, *Health or Hoax*, Sphere, 1986.

British Dietetic Association, *The Great British Diet*, Century, 1985.

British Medical Association, *Executive Health*, BMA, 1979.

Bowden, J. and Burr, R., *Food Can Damage Your Health*, Rosters, 1989.

Buckroy, Julia, *Eating Your Heart Out*, Optima, 1989.

Cannon, G. and Einzig H., *Dieting Makes You Fat*, Sphere, 1984.

Chaitow, Leon, *Candida Albicans*, Thorsons, 1985.

Chaitow, Leon, *Fatigue*, Thorsons, 1988.

Conley, Rosemary, *Hip and Thigh Diet*, Arrow, 1988.

de Vries, Jan, *Realistic Weight Control*, Mainstream, 1989.

Douglas, Cathy, *The Superwoman Trap*, Futura, 1984.

Eyton, Audrey, *The F-Plan Diet*, Penguin, 1982.

Hanssen, Maurice, *E for Additives*, Thorsons, 1987.

Holford, Patrick, *Optimum Nutrition*, Ion Press, 1992.

Holford, P. and Woods, B., *Fat Burner Diet*, Ion Press, 1992.

Jacobs, Gill, *Candida Albicans*, Macdonald Optima, 1990.

Kenton, Leslie, *10 Day Clean-up Plan*, Century Hutchinson, 1986.

Lashford, Stephanie, *The Residue Report*, Thorsons, 1981.

Lawrence, Dana, *Fighting Food*, Penguin, 1990.

London Food Commission, *Food Adulteration*, Unwin, 1988.

Maisner, Paulette, *Excuses Won't Cure You*, Unwin, 1987.

Maisner, P. and Pulling, J., *Feasting and Fasting*, Fontana, 1985.

Martlaw, G. and Silver, S., *The Pill Protection Plan*, Grapevine, 1989.

Mervyn, Leonard, *Vitamins and Minerals*, Thorsons, 1989.

Mumby, Dr Keith, *The Allergy Handbook*, Thorsons, 1993.

Orbach, Susie, *Fat is a Feminist Issue 2*, Hamlyn, 1984.

Paterson, Barbara, *The Allergy Connection*, Thorsons, 1985.

Polunin, Miriam, *The Health and Fitness Handbook*, Sphere, 1983.

Richardson, Diane, *Women and the AIDS Crisis*, Pandora, 1989.

Shaevitz, Marjorie, *The Superwoman Syndrome*, Fontana, 1985.

Solomon, Dr Henry, *The Exercise Myth*, Angus & Robertson, 1985.

Stewart, Maryon, *Beat PMT Through Diet*, Ebury Press, 1990.

Stewart, A. and Stewart M., *The Vitality Diet*, Thorsons, 1990.

Temple et al., *Food for Action*, Pelham, 1987.

Townsend, P., Black, D., Whitehead, M., *Inequalities in Health*, Penguin, 1992.

Walker, C. and Cannon, G., *The Food Scandal*, Century, 1984.

Wells, C.L., *Women, Sport and Performance*, Human Kinetics, 1985.

Wills, Judith, *A Flat Stomach in 15 Days*, Sphere, 1990.

Wilson, Dr R.C.D., *Pre-menstrual Syndrome: Diet Against It*, Foulsham, 1988.

Pamphlets, Articles, etc.

'Diet and Cardiovascular Disease', DHSS: COMA (Committee on Medical Aspects of Food Policy).

'A Discussion Paper on Proposals for Nutritional Guidelines for Health Education in Britain', prepared for NACNE by

Professor W. James et al., London, Health Education Council (now Authority), 1983.

'Healthier Eating and Your Heart', Coronary Prevention Group.

'Report on Health and Social Subjects' No. 28, HMSO, 1979.

Glossary

Abdomen Region of the lower torso containing digestive organs (stomach, intestines, etc.).

Active Taking a deliberate action.

Acute Severe, urgent symptoms with rapid onset and swift resolution.

Adrenalin Stress hormone.

Allergen Substance giving rise to an allergic reaction.

Allergy Inability to tolerate exposure to a substance.

Amino acids Protein-derived organic compounds essential to human biology.

Anecdotal Drawn from general observed experience rather than scientific study.

Appetite Desire as opposed to need to eat.

Arterial disease Degeneration of the arteries.

Arteriosclerosis Thickening and loss of elasticity of the walls of the arteries.

Asthma Chronic respiratory disorder.

Beverage Liquid refreshment.

Bloatedness Specific sudden swelling and discomfort of the abdomen associated with fluid retention.

Calories Unit of heat – in nutrition terms a unit of dietary fuel energy.

Candida *Candida albicans*, a yeast present in the bowel.

Carbohydrate Starch/sugar organic compound made up of

carbon, hydrogen and oxygen. *See* refined, complex and simple carbohydrate.

Cardiac disease Degeneration of the heart.

Cholesterol Waxy sterol compound occurring in animal tissues.

Chronic Long-term problem with low-level symptoms.

Coeliac disease Disease of the intestines.

Complementary medicine Non-orthodox treatment methods working alongside conventional medicine.

Condiment Added sauce or seasoning for food.

Congenital A condition existing from birth.

Controls A scientific sample group tested to avoid coincidences appearing in experiment results.

Diagnosis The process of discovering the source of discomfort, in this book applied to the method of discovering a programme of eating most likely to result in successful fat-loss in a specific individual.

Diet Composition of regular food intake, does not necessarily refer to a low-calorie or slimming diet.

Dietary Obtained through food intake.

Digestion Process by which food is metabolised in the body.

Eating plan An individual programme of eating (not necessarily low-calorie) aimed at alleviating specific symptoms. Low-calorie; low-fat; low-sugar; low-cholesterol; low-processing; menstrual syndrome; oral contraceptive syndrome; anti-candida; low-allergen; special requirements; vegetarian.

Eczema Allergic skin disorder.

Energy Fuel derived from calories.

Environmental Deriving from external circumstances, e.g. surroundings.

Epidemiology The study of the genesis of mass diseases.

Essential fatty acid Trace element deriving mainly from certain seeds and plants, should not be confused with fat.

Experimental The conduct of scientific investigation.

Glossary

Fibre Indigestible dietary roughage.

Flow chart Diagram used to diagnose application of correct eating plans.

Food intolerance Mild allergy.

Food sensitivity Varying allergic reaction.

Gluten A protein present in cereal grains, especially wheat.

HDL An apparently beneficial form of cholesterol.

Hunger Need for food as opposed to mere desire for food (see appetite).

Hypoglycaemia Lowered blood sugar level.

Irritable bowel Varying syndrome of intestinal symptoms including constipation and diarrhoea.

LDL A harmful form of cholesterol.

Menstrual syndrome Group of symptoms present in association with the menstrual cycle.

Metabolism The chemical progress of sustaining organic life.

Migraine Severe allergic-type headache.

Minerals Traces of metals necessary to the human metabolism.

Monounsaturate A type of fat derived from plants and seeds which remains liquid at room temperature and is thought to be neutral or beneficial to health.

NACNE National Advisory Committee on Nutrition Education.

Nutrition The process of deriving energy from dietary sources.

Obesity Overfatness of varying degrees.

Observations Points noted through scientific study, though not necessarily in experimental conditions.

Obsession An unrelenting fascination with or repeated need for some experience, akin to addiction.

Obsessive compulsive disorder Situation in which the obsession comes to dominate the sufferer's life.

Oral contraceptive Medication containing combinations of progesterone and oestrogen resulting in arrested fertility.

Orthodox Recognised and approved thinking.

Overfat Carrying too much excess fat on the body.

Overweight A confusing term generally misused to mean overfat. Weight is not a major attribute of fat. The term is strictly only applied in sports where weight is a factor in determining competitive category, e.g. horse-racing, boxing.

Oxidation Degeneration of a cell or other substance in reaction to oxygen.

Passive Experiencing without conscious effort on the part of the experiencer.

Polyunsaturate Long chain molecule fat derived from seeds and plants.

Preserving Protecting or otherwise inhibiting food from deterioration during storage by artificial or natural methods.

Processing Artificial methods of preserving and presenting foods.

Prognosis Outlook.

Protein Form of nutrient.

Pulses Dried beans, peas, lentils and other cereal seeds.

Rebound dieting Yo-yo dieting, 'Monday Syndrome', connected with reactive hypoglycaemia.

Risk factor A pre-existor which disposes a patient towards contracting a disease without being the main cause of the disease.

Saturated Short chain molecule fat derived from animals.

Slimming diet Conventional catch-all diets which are claimed to be equally successful in treating a wide range of eating/overfat problems.

Statistics Figures relating to a subject.

Stop food A food which must be cut out on a particular eating plan.

Stress Disturbance caused by environmental factors and/or emotional trauma.

Substitute food A food which may be eaten instead of a stop food, designed to give the same sort of emotional reward.

Sugar Refined carbohydrate.

Trace elements Dietary substances needed by the body in very small quantities.

Vitamins Important dietary substances needed to aid metabolic processes.

Yeast Living mould organism related to *Candida albicans*.